Communication: The Key to the Therapeutic Relationship

. . . .

Communication: The Key to the Therapeutic Relationship

Pamela McHugh Schuster, RN, PhD
Associate Professor of Nursing
Youngstown State University
Youngstown, Ohio

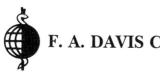 F. A. DAVIS COMPANY • Philadelphia

F. A. Davis Company
1915 Arch Street
Philadelphia, PA 19103

Printed in the United States of America

Last digit indicates print number: 10 9 8 7 6 5 4 3 2 1

Acquisitions Editor: Joanne P. DaCunha, RN, MSN
Developmental Editor: Catherine Harold
Production Editor: Jessica Howie Martin
Cover Designer: Louis J. Forgione
Cartoons: John Chlebus and Mike Damen

As new scientific information becomes available through basic and clinical research, recommended treatments and drug therapies undergo changes. The author and publisher have done everything possible to make this book accurate, up to date, and in accord with accepted standards at the time of publication. The author, editors, and publisher are not responsible for errors or omissions or for consequences from application of the book, and make no warranty, expressed or implied, in regard to the contents of the book. Any practice described in this book should be applied by the reader in accordance with professional standards of care used in regard to the unique circumstances that may apply in each situation. The reader is advised always to check product information (package inserts) for changes and new information regarding dose and contraindications before administering any drug. Caution is especially urged when using new or infrequently ordered drugs.

Library of Congress Cataloging-in-Publication Data

Schuster, Pamela A., 1953
    Communicaton: the key to the therapeutic relationship/by Pamela A. Schuster.
        p. cm.
    Includes bibliographical references and index.
    ISBN 0-8036-0469-6
    1. Nurse and patient. 2. Interpersonal communication. 3. Communication in
nursing. I. Title.
    [DNLM: 1. Nurse-Patient Relations. 2. Communication Nurses'
Instruction. 3. Nursing Care—psychology. WY 87 S395c 1999]
    RT86.3.S525 1999
    810.73'06'99—9c21
    DNLM/DLC   99-38640
    for Library of Congress   CIP

This book is dedicated to my husband Fred and children Luke, Leeanna, Patty, and Isaac.

Preface

· · · · · · · · · · ·

Nursing students and faculty members wholeheartedly agree that a student's ability to communicate therapeutically and form a therapeutic relationship is fundamental to the entire nursing care delivery process. Therapeutic communication is critical to accurate assessment of patient care situations and intervention with patients. However, merely having a conceptual understanding of therapeutic communication has little to do with applying its principles to the daily clinical situations that nursing students encounter.

Everyone communicates, but not everyone knows how to do so therapeutically. This book was written for nursing students who are having their first encounters with patients, to serve as a guide to better therapeutic communication when interacting with patients. While working with fundamentals and medical-surgical nursing students in multiple clinical settings for the past 17 years, I have observed hundreds of students who expressed anxiety about what to do or say to patients to establish and maintain a therapeutic relationship. All of the examples used in this book come from the numerous student-patient and staff-patient interactions I have observed in clinical settings.

Communication: The Key to the Therapeutic Relationship has been written especially for novice students to fill the void between the single chapter on communication usually found in fundamental books and advanced books on communication such as psychiatric mental health texts. This book contains a succinct fundamental overview of essential therapeutic communication theories and techniques with real-life examples of how to apply therapeutic techniques in clinical situations.

This book is intended to be user friendly and is written in a format that is easy to read and comprehend, with the incorporation of chapter objectives, chapter summaries, and bibliographies for further reading. There are numerous real-life examples, some humorous and some serious. Because humor is an important aspect of communication, cartoons are used to illustrate important concepts. End-of-chapter exercises are provided to allow practice of therapeutic communication skills.

Communication: The Key to the Therapeutic Relationship was written to accompany basic fundamental and medical-surgical texts and to be used to help nursing students develop comprehensive holistic plans of care. Nursing students need a reference book to assist in the development of these plans using effective communication techniques to intervene in the psychosocial care of patients as well as using protocols and procedures for their physical care. The book is also intended as a psychosocial communication intervention reference in clinical settings.

The first four chapters involve application of theories of communication to the assessment of crucial factors that affect communication processes. These chapters focus on the interaction of the emotional, social, cultural, and physical components of each person in the communication process, both the patient and the student nurse. Thus, not only must patients be assessed and understood regarding what they are trying to communicate, but students must focus on self-assessment, self-understanding, and self-monitoring during interactions with patients. Self-assessment quizzes are incorporated to provide insight into personal communication patterns and beliefs.

In Chapter 1, the framework is developed and an overview is provided for the rest of the book. Basic communication and therapeutic communication are defined and described. This first chapter is intended to give students a better understanding of communication processes in stressful healthcare environments and the emotional reactions of people in healthcare settings. Emphasis is placed on the typical reactions of both patient and nurse to stressful situations.

Chapters 2 and 3 deal with the importance of gender and cultural issues, as well as with self-esteem and body image issues for patient and nurse. These factors are very important to assess and understand for effective therapeutic communication. Chapter 4 delves into the specific emotional reactions of people when they are ill, which further complicate communication processes.

Chapters 5 through 10 are each written to provide information on using specific therapeutic communication interventions to work effectively with patients in accomplishing mutual health-related goals. Chapter 5 explains how to use the communication intervention techniques of assertiveness, responsiveness, and empathy. Chapters 6 and 7 describe communication interventions using touch and humor, and Chapter 8 tells what to do when the patient is sad and cries. Chapter 9 covers principles of patient education integrating the use of therapeutic communication techniques. Chapter 10 is about helping patients use the basic problem-solving process and guiding patients to make decisions using therapeutic communication techniques.

Therapeutic communication is one of the cornerstones of all nursing practice in any setting. No matter what your current level of expertise as a communicator, this book can be a guide to becoming more therapeutic.

I wish to acknowledge and thank my editors Joanne DaCunha and Catherine Harold for their support and encouragement throughout the writing and production of this book. I especially want to thank the artists John Chlebus and Mike Damen for the wonderful cartoons they contributed to this book. Humor is a very important component of all aspects of communication, and serves to lighten up everyone's lives. Cartoons make learning about therapeutic communication enjoyable. A special thanks to my family and friends who are always there for me. They provide me with all kinds of outlets from work, and I love them all very much.

Pamela McHugh Schuster

A Note about Usage

. . . .

To avoid both sexism and the constant repetition of "he or she," "his or her," and so forth, masculine and feminine pronouns are used alternately throughout the text.

Reviewers

. . . .

M. Star Mahara, RN, MSN(C)
Instructor, Nursing Programs
School of Nursing
University College of the Cariboo
Kamloops, B.C., Canada

Susan A. Newfield, RN, PhD, CS
Assistant Professor
School of Nursing
West Virginia University Health Sciences Center
Morgantown, West Virginia

Dona Pardo, RN, PhD
Coordinator, Continuing Education
College of Nursing
University of Arizona
Tucson, Arizona

Dolores S. Patrinos, RN, MA
College of Allied Health, Department of Nursing
Temple University
Philadelphia, Pennsylvania

Kaye Ronsman, RN, MSN
Geriatric Nurse Practitioner
Veterans Administration Hospital
Tucson, Arizona

Contents

. . . .

Therapeutic Communication: The Foundation of Professional Practice

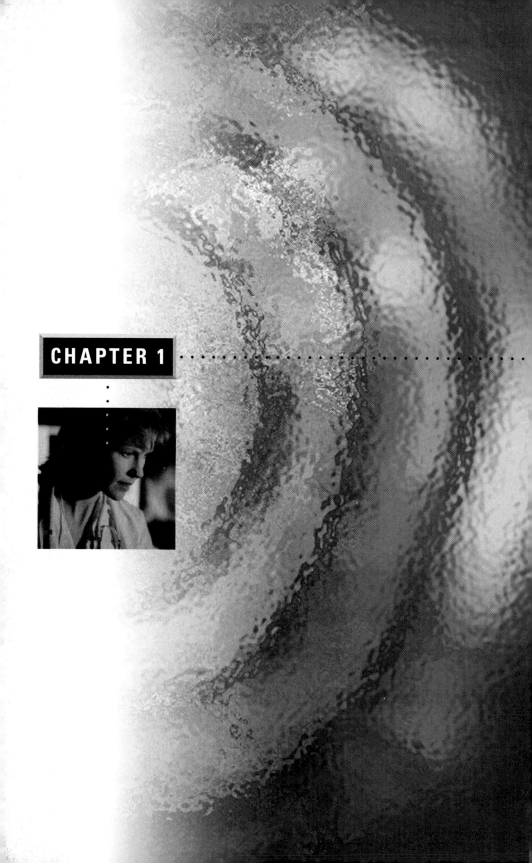

CHAPTER 1

Therapeutic Communication: The Foundation of Professional Practice

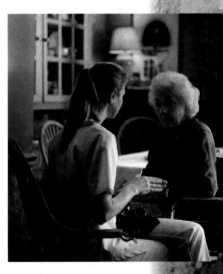

Chapter Objectives

AFTER READING THIS CHAPTER,
YOU WILL BE ABLE TO:

1. Compare and contrast the definitions of communication and therapeutic communication.
2. List the goals of therapeutic communication.
3. Identify the basic elements of communication from telecommunication and psychotherapy theories.
4. List four major principles of therapeutic communication.
5. Describe the "Life Fields" communication theory as it relates to communication in healthcare settings.
6. Identify communication distortion factors in healthcare environments.
7. Discuss the importance of recognizing physical and emotional responses to healthcare situations.
8. Describe the five universal communication styles that people use to respond to stressful situations.

HAVE YOU EVER WONDERED WHY IT'S EASY TO TALK TO SOME PEOPLE BUT difficult to talk to others? Naturally, there are many reasons. You'll learn about some of the most important ones in this book. And you'll learn how to help yourself become a person who's easy to talk to, a person your patients can trust, a person who makes the most of patients' goals and objectives—in short, a good therapeutic communicator.

No matter what your level of current expertise as a communicator, this book was written for you to use as a guide for becoming more therapeutic in your interactions with patients. This chapter introduces the process of therapeutic communication, especially as it applies to professional nursing. Chapters 2 through 4 expand on personal characteristics that influence how people communicate, such as gender, culture, self-esteem, and emotional reactions. Chapters 5 through 8 focus on specific nursing communication interventions, including basic facilitation techniques, empathy, touch, and the therapeutic use of humor and tears. The last two chapters discuss the integration of therapeutic communication into patient education and the process of helping patients solve problems.

Conversations between a nurse and a patient need to get to the essence of the problem. Mutual goals need to be established and a plan of care designed and implemented in the briefest possible time. Patients and family members must feel that you understand their physical and emotional needs and that you hear what they are trying to say to you. You must clearly and therapeutically communicate back to the patient that the message sent was correctly received, and then also clearly and therapeutically communicate what needs to be done next to manage the current situation.

Is it possible to accomplish all this in a timely manner and have the patient and family exclaim about the wonderful care they received and how well they were treated by healthcare providers? It *is* possible if you know how to communicate therapeutically. Please take note of the word *therapeutic*. Everyone communicates, but not everyone knows how to be therapeutic. Before you can get there yourself, you'll need to understand basic communication.

Basic Communication Theory: Elements of Messages

How well have you learned to communicate? Since infancy, you have been communicating. You started with nonverbal behaviors and loud crying. In response, your parents or caretakers tried to discern and meet your needs, and you stopped crying and settled down. Some of you stopped crying and settled down more quickly than others; anyone who has raised more than one child can verify that fact.

As you grew up, you learned more about how to communicate your wants and needs. You learned how to influence others, how to ask questions to obtain information, and how to elicit a response from other people. However, some of you have learned how to communicate better than others. Some of you get what you want more often than others do. Some of you are more satisfied with your personal relationships.

At times, all of us have difficulty understanding the words or behaviors of others. Sometimes all of us feel that we aren't understood. In either case, the communication process has broken down. Communication is the use of words and behaviors to construct, send, and interpret messages. It is a process by which one individual may affect another through written, verbal, and nonverbal means.[1]

Factors that make communication successful and factors that cause it to break down have been studied for many years, with theoretical roots in the fields of telecommunication and psychotherapy.[2,3] The purpose of any theory or model is to help us make sense of what is happening around us. This basic theoretical model of the communication process is shown on page 5. Communication in this theoretical model is simply defined as the interactive process of transmitting a message or idea. The interactive process occurs between two or more persons. The sender must clearly encode a message using both verbal

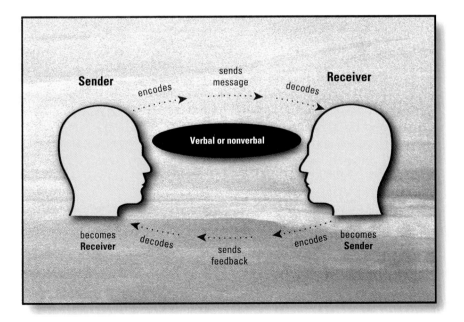

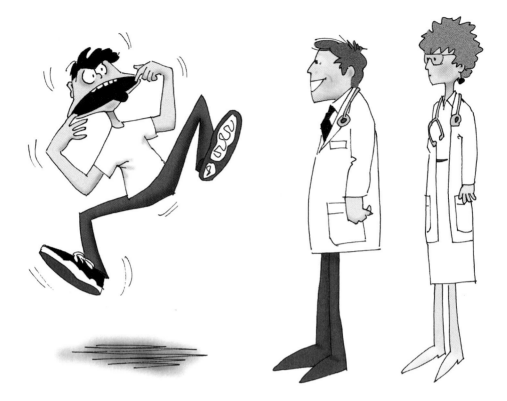

and nonverbal behaviors, the message must be clearly transmitted through the environment, and the receiver must correctly decode the message sent. The message has then been sent and received, but has it been received correctly? Has the receiver really understood the message? At this point, the sender can't be sure.

Therefore, the next important step to complete the communication process is for the receiver to become a sender and encode a feedback message that goes back through the environment to be decoded by the original sender, who is now the receiver. In other words, the person sending the original message must receive acknowledgment from the original receiver to confirm that the message has been understood.

For communication to be successful, a message must be verified. As depicted in the cartoon on page 6, feedback is essential for you to know where you stand with the other person, once you have sent them a message. A humorous saying by an unknown author summarizes the need to clearly send and receive messages: "I know you believe you understand what you think I said, but I am not sure you realize that what you heard is not what I meant."

Defining Therapeutic Communication

Therapeutic communication involves the use of carefully selected communication interventions to help patients and families overcome stress and adjust to the unalterable. When you use therapeutic communication effectively, you help patients clearly identify their problems and needs by helping them express themselves effectively. You can also use therapeutic communication to help patients examine their options and develop a plan to correct the problem at hand. Therapeutic communication is the foundation of professional practice, and you must learn to do it well.

NURSE-PATIENT COMMUNICATIONS

Nurse-patient communications differ from the communication that takes place between you and other members of the healthcare team, and it differs from your day-to-day communications outside the healthcare system. The difference is that patients have unmet safety and security needs that your friends and colleagues don't. Specifically, patients are in vulnerable positions because they are no longer capable of independent self-care, and they're often dependent on healthcare providers whom they don't know personally. Patients seek the assistance of healthcare providers to prevent health problems, to detect and treat acute and chronic health problems, and when no more can be done, to find a way to die peacefully. Health concerns are very personal and private matters to resolve. Managing health concerns can become frustrating and upsetting to patients and families and can affect the way in which they communicate.

A primary aspect of your role is to communicate therapeutically to direct the patient toward the attainment of his or her health goals and objectives. The patient's health outcomes may depend largely on your clinical knowledge and your ability to communicate in the healthcare setting.

The flowchart on page 8 contrasts the outcomes of nursing communications that are therapeutic versus those that are not therapeutic. In therapeutic communication, you develop a collaborative relationship with your patient and establish mutual goals and objectives. If communication is not therapeutic, conflict develops in the nurse-patient relationship over goals and objectives.

From the moment you and a patient first meet, a reaction occurs as you interact and attempt to establish mutual goals, objectives, and a plan of action to solve health-related problems. As shown in the flowchart, the nurse goes into a patient care situation with a precon-

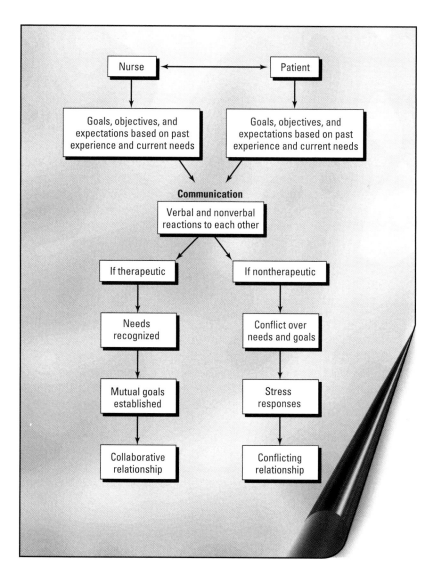

ceived set of goals and objectives that he believes need to be achieved for an optimal health outcome. The nurse also has a preconceived set of ideas about how he should act and how the patient should act in the situation. Each patient and family member also has a preconceived set of perceptions and expectations about the healthcare system, about how a patient should act, and about how healthcare providers should act. The patient has her own set of goals and objectives that she believes must be achieved for an optimal health outcome. You and your patient may or may not have the same goals and objectives related to health outcomes.

During your first and subsequent encounters with a patient, you'll communicate to establish mutual goals and objectives regarding problems, and you'll develop plans for solving those problems. The patient may have different ideas than you do about what the problems are, as well as different ideas about what should be done and how things should be done to solve those problems. If you and your patient agree on what the problems are and you have a similar set of expectations about health goals, objectives, and plans to correct problems, then there should be very little conflict between you and the patient. However, differing ideas about the problem and what to do about it may lead to conflict. Consequently, you and the patient will both feel stress.

To understand your role in responding to these conflicting perspectives between you and a patient, consider the following example. Suppose your goal is to prevent the complications of immobility for a particular elderly patient in a nursing home. You go into his room to get him out of bed for breakfast. The patient acts very sleepy and says, "I don't want to get up. Let me sleep." You know that trays are coming in 20 minutes and that the patient is scheduled to be in physical therapy in an hour. Do you assert your authority and tell the patient that he has to get up right away? This may upset the patient because he feels that you're treating him as though he were a child and you were the authority figure. You would not be respecting his needs or desires. On the other hand, should you let him sleep? If you do, your clinical faculty and physical therapist won't be happy with you.

What should you do? The answer is to go to where the patient is. Pick up on what the patient says is important to him. This person wants sleep, which is a very basic physical need. So you say, "You're tired today. How did you sleep last night?"

He responds with, "The patient across the hall was making noise all night."

"I guess the staff should have passed out ear plugs last night," you say, in a slightly joking tone.

The patient smiles a little, and says, "You can say that again!"

Now that you've recognized that the patient has an unmet need for sleep and you've communicated that you understand his need, you can once again direct him toward his mobility goals. Say something like, "Breakfast trays are coming in 20 minutes and you have an appointment in physical therapy in an hour. Would you like 5 minutes more to sleep now, and then I'll be come to get you up? There's also a period between therapy and lunch when you can take a nap when you get back. I'll hang a *Do not disturb* sign on your door if you'd like." You must let the patient know that his need will be met. Then you can negotiate mutual goals, and the patient will most likely cooperate.

Once you negotiate a solution with the patient, however, you must follow through and be true to your word. You told him he could have a nap, so make sure that he gets one. That way, the patient will learn that he can trust you and that you're someone he can count on to look out for him. This example illustrates therapeutic techniques being used to recognize the patient's needs, put the patient at ease by establishing a trusting relationship, and enlist the patient's cooperation in establishing mutual goals and objectives that will lead to optimal health outcomes.

COMMUNICATION IN PROFESSIONAL RELATIONSHIPS

To be effective as a professional nurse, you also need to know how and when to communicate with other members of the healthcare team. You won't be using therapeutic communication because the objectives of your communication with other professionals differ from the objectives of your communication with patients.

You need not establish a therapeutic relationship with other healthcare providers. Instead, you should develop a formal, collegial relationship with them. Working together, you and other healthcare providers will help patients identify and solve their health-related problems. In most cases, your role will be to describe clearly patient assessment data relevant to other healthcare providers so that they can better perform their roles for each patient.

The following example outlines a clinical situation that involves a combination of therapeutic communication with a patient and professional communication with a colleague, in this case a surgeon. A patient came to a surgical center for knee replacement surgery and needed to be ready to go to surgery in 2 hours. A nurse goes into the patient's room to complete an admission assessment and begins asking the routine questions needed to complete the form. Some of these questions are personal, and some refer to family relationships. The nurse had planned to start at the top of the form and work through the questions to the bottom.

However, the patient begins to grow visibly upset by these routine questions and says, "These questions are irrelevant and none of your business." It was only the nurse's second day on the preoperative unit, and when she performed the assessment the day before, the patient just answered the questions without a problem. So why was this patient reluctant to answer them?

In this situation, the patient and the nurse had different sets of expectations. The nurse wanted to get the form completed efficiently because the information on it was needed to ensure quality care. Plus, it was hospital policy that all patients have a thorough assessment before surgery. However, the nurse made the mistake of not *first* assessing the patient's emotional state and identifying his expectations and needs. It would have been better to save the routine questions and start by asking, "How are you doing today?" while looking him in the eye and carefully evaluating his verbal and nonverbal behaviors. Had the nurse started with that question, the example would have gone much differently. The patient would have immediately asked, "Do you know how much bleeding I'll have after surgery?"

The nurse could then have said, "You seem concerned about bleeding. Some bleeding is expected, and you will be transfused with your own blood that drains from the wound."

The patient responds, "I have a friend who had the same surgery I'm having, and he started bleeding and had to be taken back to surgery. What if that happens to me?"

Now the nurse knows what the patient is really concerned about: his need to be physically safe and his doubts about the safety of the procedure itself. With that information in hand, the nurse could say, "Since your friend was sent back to surgery, it sounds like he had complications that aren't typical of most knee surgery procedures. We rarely send patients back to surgery, although it does happen once in a while. Would you like to talk with your surgeon to clarify what will be done and the potential complications of the procedure? I could call her and let her know you'd like to discuss the procedure more."

The nurse calls in other healthcare providers as necessary to meet goals and objectives, depending on the roles of those other health care providers in the situation. In the example, the nurse knows that it's the surgeon's role to describe the procedure to the patient, outline its risks and possible complications, and obtain the patient's informed consent. When the patient agrees, the nurse calls the surgeon, who says that she'll be up to talk in 30 minutes. Now the nurse can go back to the patient and say, "The doctor said she would be up to see you in 30 minutes. In the meantime, I have some routine questions that we ask everyone before they have surgery. Can we work on this until she gets here?" The patient is now more likely to cooperate with the assessment.

Frequently, you'll use therapeutic communication to identify patients' healthcare concerns and needs. However, it's important to recognize that you do not need to meet personally each of the needs you uncover. Indeed, it's important to know when to refer the problems you identify to other healthcare providers, in this case the physician. As a patient educator, you can talk in general terms about a procedure and what usually happens. You can reinforce the surgeon's earlier explanation to the patient. But if the patient needs additional specific information about a procedure, as in this case, it would not be your role to provide it. Instead, it would be the surgeon's role. You use professional communication techniques each time you inform an appropriate professional about patient needs to enable that professional to perform the required service or role.

The nurse in this example used therapeutic communication to identify the basic human need for physical safety, and she used professional communication when asking the surgeon to come and clarify the procedure and its potential complications. She was then able to complete the routine assessment paperwork required by the hospital before the 2-hour deadline for the patient's surgery.

Principles of Therapeutic Communication

To provide truly therapeutic communication, you'll want to adhere to the following set of principles based on classic research on the principles of communication.[2-5]

SOLICIT FEEDBACK

Verify all messages by paying careful attention to all feedback (responses) given by the patient receiving your message. Likewise, make a conscious effort to provide feedback when you're the one receiving a message.

For example, if you're receiving a message, you should verify what you thought you heard the sender say. Successful communication requires that the mutual meaning of thoughts, feelings, or ideas be shared between two or more people. If you consistently verify the messages you send and receive, you'll have a much better chance of sharing mutual meanings.

OBSERVE BODY LANGUAGE

Pay close attention to the nonverbal messages, or body language, of the person with whom you're communicating. For example, suppose someone is trying to say something to you during a face-to-face encounter. The face is the most expressive part of the body, so you'll want to watch the person's expressions carefully. Do his eyes and mouth register fear, anger, surprise, pride, boredom, sadness, and happiness? As the cartoon on page 13 illustrates, you must become especially good at interpreting facial expressions and other nonverbal behaviors as you talk with patients, family members, and other professionals—everyone really.

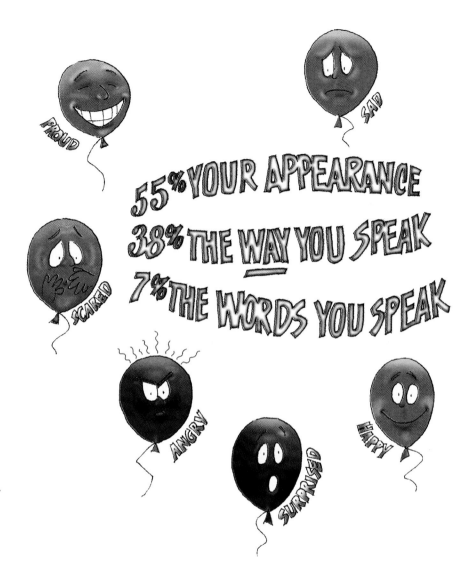

Besides facial expressions, nonverbal communication also involves body movements. How you move your hands, how high or low you hang your head, and how you stand and sit and walk communicate something to anyone who looks at you. You can use your knowledge of these body movements to help corroborate or cast doubt on your patients' verbal messages. Also keep in mind that nonverbal behavior can be less consciously controlled than verbal behavior and that actions do indeed speak louder than words.

ASSESS APPEARANCE

Your physical appearance, including the clothes you wear, also affects communication. For example, as a student nurse, you are told you must look "professional" during clinical courses. Professional may be defined as well groomed and wearing clothes that are neat, clean, and pressed regardless of whether you are wearing a lab coat, uniform, or street clothes. Clothing that is businesslike and practical is ideal. Professional attire does not have to be expensive, trendy, or elegant.

Picture yourself in a comfortable pair of jeans and a sweatshirt versus a pair of dress pants, blouse or shirt, and a white lab coat with a stethoscope in your pocket. Jeans may be fine for a lecture course but not if you want to look professional. You must be very conscious of the message your appearance gives to your patients and colleagues. Also, take note of the appearance of the person with whom you are trying to communicate. Her physical appearance will give you clues about her physical and emotional state.

RESPOND TO THE REAL MESSAGE

Have you heard the expression, "It's not what you say, but how you say it?" It's true. The tone of the voice is more important than the words you use to communicate a message. For example, say you walk into a room to do a morning assessment and find the patient pacing back and forth. When you ask how he's doing today, he responds with a shaky voice that's hardly audible, "I'm fine, thank you."

By assessing the patient's nonverbal behaviors, however, you can clearly see that he's not fine. So, ignoring his words and responding to his nonverbal cues and tone of voice, you move in closer to the patient and, with concern in your voice, you say, "You're pacing and your voice is shaky. What's the matter?"

The patient responds with, "I'm very concerned about how my tests are going to turn out. I just know I have cancer."

Now you're getting somewhere closer to how the patient is really doing today. As you attempt to decode the true meaning of a message, focus on how well the person's nonverbal behavior, tone of voice, and words match up. If the person's nonverbal cues and tone of voice don't match the words he speaks, you'll want to respond to the nonverbals and tone, not the words. Remember always to verify the message, and rely most heavily on the nonverbal cues and tone as you formulate a response. The spoken words have the least importance in helping you clearly decipher a message.

Research by Mehrabian on nonverbal communication showed that appearance and body language account for 55 percent of the way in which a message is interpreted. The tone of voice accounts for 38 percent of a message. The actual words spoken have the least amount of importance in the interpretation of a message, accounting for only 7 percent of the total message delivered.[4,5] One sign of a good communicator is that the nonverbal behaviors, tone of voice, and words match the message.

Distinguishing the Patient's View from Your Own

To be therapeutic, you must aim to understand a situation from the patient's viewpoint. How does the patient perceive the situation, and how is it similar to or different from the perceptions you hold as the healthcare provider? The Life Fields Theory offers key factors to help you understand your patient's viewpoint and assess your own viewpoints. This theory implies that it is important for healthcare providers to develop self-awareness through self-appraisal of one's own culturally derived feelings, beliefs, attitudes, and values. In other words, you must evaluate your own life experiences, social and environmental backgrounds, gender issues, and self-concept that you bring into the interaction with the patient.

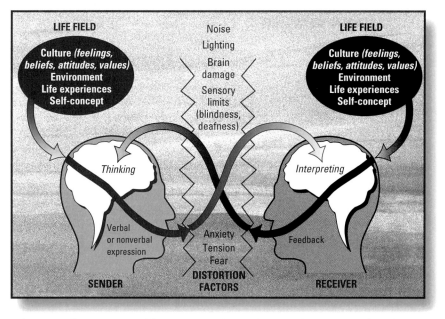

Grimes, J and Burns, E: Health Assessment in Nursing Practice. Jones and Bartlett, Sudbury, Massachusetts, 1998. www.jbpub.com. Reprinted with permission.

This theory has its roots in the field of perceptual psychology and has been adapted to depict key factors for consideration in nurse-patient interactions.[6,7] It shows two people communicating, taking into consideration the Life Fields—or psychological, social, and cultural experiences—of both people involved in the exchange. The diagram on page 15 depicts important concepts from the Life Fields Theory.

In general, the better the match between the life fields of the patient and the nurse, the easier it is to communicate. Suppose it was a stressful busy day on the oncology unit, and four patients lay dying, surrounded by family members. They were from four different religious backgrounds: Catholic, Hindu, Jewish, and Muslim. If you had your choice of assignment, which one would you take? You would probably pick the one that was most similar to your own background because it would be easiest to understand the customs, practices, and beliefs of the dying person and the surrounding family members. It would be much more difficult to anticipate the spiritual needs of a person and family from a culture unfamiliar to you.

In a second example, a patient comes into the surgical center and has to be in the operating room by 7:30 AM. Two strangers, you (a nurse), the other (a patient), meet for the first time. You use therapeutic communication and pay very careful attention to the verbal and nonverbal messages the patient sends. You introduce yourself, shake the patient's hand, and smile. The patient smiles back. You appear to be off to a good start based on the patient's response, otherwise known as feedback. What if the patient said "Hello" but didn't smile and looked down at the floor without making eye contact? Now what? You started out the same way both times with an introduction, handshake, and smile. So what happened?

Although you started out with the same approach, each patient responded differently. Patient responses can differ based on a number of factors. The patient's life experiences up to the point when you meet in a healthcare setting guide her response in the healthcare situation. For example, what has the patient's experience been with the healthcare system and healthcare providers? How familiar is she with the healthcare environment? Has the patient ever had surgery before? Has she ever been hospitalized? In addition, social and cultural influences passed down through generations of the patient's family guide her feelings, beliefs, attitudes, and values. Likewise, they'll affect her response to you. Age and gender also influence each patient's responses, as do the effects of the person's self-concept.

Also keep in mind that the same procedure can mean very different things to the patient, depending on the underlying reason for it. Consider two 40-year-old patients having hysterectomies because uterine fibroids are causing them to have painful menstruation and heavy bleeding each month. One patient has four children and is looking forward to the pain relief the surgery is likely to bring. The other patient has not been able to conceive despite years of effort. Which one will return your smile as you enter the room, and which will be looking down at the floor?

Each of these factors affects verbal and nonverbal expressions as a nurse and patient meet and react to each other for the first time. These factors are powerful forces that direct the way each of you think. Also, they influence how you both send and receive messages. This is why nurses are required to take courses in psychology, sociology, and philosophy. You need to understand why patients behave the way they do in general and then apply that knowledge to the way a specific person is responding in a healthcare situation. That's part of what makes nursing challenging and interesting.

The bottom line is that any two patients scheduled for the same surgery are likely to respond differently—perhaps very differently—to the situation. It's up to you as the nurse to assess those responses and guide each patient to the most optimal health outcomes possible.

Communication Distortion Factors

Also described in the Life Fields Theory are situation distortion factors that are very important to consider when attempting to communicate therapeutically. Distortion factors interfere with clear communication. They include environmental conditions, physical conditions, and emotional stresses that block the sending and receiving of clear messages. For example, noise is an environmental consideration. Too much noise when you're trying to carry on a conversation with a patient is disruptive. Lack of privacy is another example of an environmental hindrance to communication.

A patient with physical problems, such as sensory deficits resulting from blindness, deafness, or brain damage, will present different communication challenges. Also, such common physical problems as pain, hunger, and sleep deprivation will impair communication. In addition, the emotions of anxiety, tension, and fear are key distortion factors common to *all* healthcare situations. Virtually all patients and family members feel some degree of anxiety, tension, or fear as they face the stress of managing a healthcare situation and interacting with healthcare providers.

When either person in a communication interaction is under stress, communication becomes more difficult. In healthcare environments, there are plenty of reasons for everyone to feel stressed: patients, families, and even the healthcare providers themselves. The patients and families need to change their lives, at least temporarily, sometimes permanently, to adapt to health problems and related needs. Healthcare providers are typically rushed because they're short-staffed in this age of workplace redesign. Healthcare providers need to move on quickly to the next patient or to the seemingly unending pile of paperwork. We need to "do more with less" is a common slogan in many healthcare settings.

Stress, whether physical or emotional, causes the body to respond with a fight-or-flight reaction to the stressor. The theory of stress and seminal research on the fight-or-flight reaction has been credited to the world-renowned psychologist Hans Selye.[8] During the fight-or-flight reaction, hormones are released that increase blood pressure, pulse, and breathing. The pupils dilate and the palms sweat. A person's perception of environmental events creates stress, which leads to physiological reactions, with emotional and behavioral consequences.

This response occurs whenever a person's basic needs aren't met. Basic needs that could be threatened during stressful situations have been categorized by Maslow, who developed the basic human needs theory.[9] He categorized basic human needs as safety and security, love and belonging, self-esteem, and physiological needs. Some or all of these categories of needs may be threatened as a result of a health problem.

When basic human needs are threatened in any situation, health-oriented or otherwise, people react emotionally and behaviorally. The feelings that accompany the situation are very uncomfortable. The person feels anxious, nervous, and tense. He may be irritable, and he may not sleep well, get headaches, or become nauseated. It's human nature to do something to relieve these feelings of stress and anxiety. For example, the person could talk, laugh, or cry to release stressful feelings.

It is important not only to understand how patients and family members respond to the stress of a healthcare setting but also to understand your own typical response pattern when you're under stress. Healthcare situations can be very stressful for you, the nurse, as well as for patients and their families.

Remember for a moment what you feel like when someone says or does something that greatly upsets you. What are your typical verbal and nonverbal behaviors in response? What do you do to help reduce the stress you feel? Do you get angry or cry? Do you try to reason with the person who is upsetting you? Do you raise your voice? Do you remain silent and just walk away? Everyone has developed patterns of communicating under stress; you have, too.

After recognizing your typical behavior patterns under stress, you'll need to consider whether you should change any of those behaviors and develop behaviors that are more therapeutic. When interacting with patients and their families in stressful situations, it's up to you to remain in control of your verbal and nonverbal behaviors to be able to respond effectively and carry out your role. If you lose control, communication will be blocked and the emotional situation will deteriorate.

Understanding Physical and Emotional Responses

Nurses must know how to analyze and intervene in response to the physical responses of patients in healthcare settings. For example, when a patient is in labor, you must know how to attach and interpret the fetal monitor. If the baby shows signs of distress, you'll need to position the mother, start oxygen, start an intravenous line, and prepare for emergency delivery, if necessary. Obviously, when it comes to physical care for a patient, knowing what to do and how to do it is essential to your success as a nurse. Analyzing and intervening properly requires a knowledge of anatomy, physiology, physical assessment, and clinical procedures.

Just as important, however, is your ability to analyze, understand, and intervene in response to the emotional conditions of patients and their families in healthcare situations. Analyzing and intervening with emotional responses is another primary goal of nursing care, and it requires a knowledge of therapeutic communication. For example, every mother wonders if she and her child are going to make it through the delivery. Even the most rational pregnant woman, a woman who remembers that thousands of babies are born daily and that the odds favor everything coming out fine, may have some doubts that cause her tension and anxiety.

Near the end of labor, the woman has painful contractions that may cause her to lose control and begin to cry. She may become short-tempered and snap at her partner or at you because of her pain and anxiety. She may wonder if labor will ever end. To communicate with this anxious, laboring woman, speak slowly, clearly, and calmly as you provide pain control measures and help the woman breathe properly.

You also can use a communication technique called anticipatory guidance to help the patient through each contraction so the patient can cooperate and regain emotional control. In anticipatory guidance, you give a patient information that prevents her from misinterpreting a painful event and helps her understand the experience, thus reducing anxiety.[10] In this situation, you'd provide anticipatory guidance by guiding the woman though each contraction, giving specific directions and demonstrating what should be done as needed. At the same time, you would offer reassurance that everything is progressing normally, that fetal heart rate patterns show that the baby is doing well, and that the baby will be there soon.

Nurses work very hard to promote optimal physical and emotional outcomes. As a nurse, you must know what to say to patients as you administer physical care so that you can also ease the emotional stress that the patient feels. Healthcare settings are often both physically and emotionally threatening. By easing the patient's emotional stress, you enable her to cope effectively with the situation.

When you find yourself in a difficult communication situation in which emotions are tense, therapeutic communication can help facilitate optimal outcomes. In the labor and delivery scene recounted above, a calm voice tone, deliberate behaviors, and anticipatory guidance helped the patient deal with her emotional response to labor. In contrast, if a patient doesn't feel understood, or if she perceives messages incorrectly, she'll continue to feel anxious, tense, and fearful.

Patients feel threatened when they believe they are not understood or when they don't understand what's happening. If you fail to intervene early in such a situation and effectively deal with physical and emotional responses, patients and families can become very distressed. When that happens, it can become very challenging to assess, plan care for, and implement care for the distressed patient. Any time a patient is acting distressed, you should assume that her needs are not being met, and you should thoroughly assess the situation using therapeutic communication techniques.

Universal Responses to Stress

Virginia Satir has researched and developed a theory of five universal communication styles that people use to respond to stressful situations.[11,12] You must learn to recognize each of these communication styles. They're introduced in this chapter, but you'll find them again in other chapters, where the focus is on therapeutic communication interventions for each communication style. The cartoon characters on page 21 are used to represent typical responses when any of us are under stress. Satir has characterized the typical responses as Blamer, Placater, Computer, Distracter, and Leveler.

BLAMER

To illustrate, let's imagine you are a nurse going into the room of a Blamer to complete the morning assessment. You gently wake the patient, but much to your surprise, the patient starts pointing his fin-

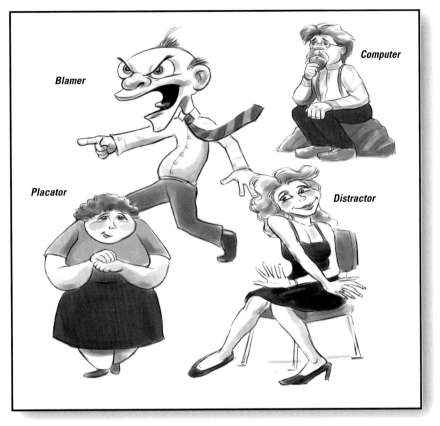

Satir, V: The New Peoplemaking Science and Behavior Books. Mountain View, 1988.

ger and loudly says, "Nobody cares what I want lying here in this bed!" and "You always come to check my blood pressure when I'm sleeping. Can't you see I'm sleeping? What's wrong with you?" All you did was to wake him to do the morning assessment that had to be done because he had surgery less than 24 hours ago. You never even met him before. He could be characterized as an aggressive bully of a person.

Characteristic of a Blamer are accusatory "you" statements, sarcasm, put-downs, expressions of superiority, and loaded words intended to start fights. The person's voice may be tense and loud or deadly quiet. His eyes may be narrowed and cold, staring, and not really "seeing" you. His posture may be stiff and rigid, with his hands on his hips. Blamers may have clenched fists, pound their fists, point a finger, and make abrupt gestures. The Blamer may interrupt, yell, call names, demand, give orders, ignore people, hang up on phone conversations, and walk away when someone is talking.

PLACATER

Then there's the Placater. You go into the next room, where you ask the patient if she has decided on the rehabilitation center that she'd like to be transferred to because she needs extensive physical therapy. She had a bad fall and broke her hip. Her family can't take care of her at home until she can do more for herself.

When you ask the question, the patient fidgets and picks at her fingernails. With a pleading look in her eyes and a soft watery voice, she says "um, I don't care . . . er, what do you think? My son wants me to go to Parkside, but then my daughter says I should go to Hillsville by her home, I mean, I'm sorry, I don't know what to do."

This person—a Placater—has a hard time coming to the point and making decisions. She may beat around the bush, issue numerous apologies, and stumble to say what she means. She is frightened of offending or angering anyone. Her eyes may be downcast, looking away, or pleading. Her posture is stooped, she may nod her head excessively, and she may be leaning for support. The person's hand gestures are fidgety or fluttery; she may wring her hands or pick at her fingernails. Other characteristic behaviors for a Placater include saying yes when she really means no, going along with others when she really doesn't want to, apologizing for things she didn't do, deciding that she can't do something before she's even tried it, and denying compliments.

COMPUTER

Out in the hall, you run into the patient's son, a Computer. You say, "Your mother is upset about where she should go for rehabilitation. She seems to be torn between the place you believe is best and the place your sister feels is best."

He replies with a monotone, matter-of-fact voice, "There's a simple solution to the problem. No rational person would need to get upset about it." The Computer doesn't want his feelings known and resists discussing them when asked. He doesn't like to show or discuss any form of emotion, usually out of fear that doing so is a sign of weakness. This person is quiet, aloof, reserved, and withdrawn. His tone of voice is quiet and monotonous. He tries to remain calm and matter of fact, no matter what happens around him. His face and eyes are expressionless. His posture is closed; he may cross his arms and legs and hold himself stiffly upright. He tends to deny his own feelings and has difficulty responding when others express their feelings to him.

DISTRACTER

Just then, the patient's daughter, the Distracter, approaches you in the hallway. You explain that her mother is upset about where she should go for rehabilitation. She turns to her brother, points a finger at him and says, "You always want things your way!" Then she turns to you with quiet, downcast eyes and says, "Whatever Mother wants, I really don't care. There should be an easy answer to the problem."

A Distracter jumps from one mode to another, following her urges about what she wants to say. She combines the Blamer, Placater, and Computer, continuously shifting modes, talking nervously, and making little sense. She expends lots of energy but doesn't focus on the problem or how to solve it.

LEVELER

The Leveler communicates with a sincere yet direct approach to manage conflict in stressful situations. The Leveler can respond effectively to various communication styles. Nurses must learn how to level in patient care situations and during communications with other healthcare professionals. Leveling is also known as assertive communication, which is the primary focus of Chapter 5.

To manage conflict in stressful situations, use a clear, firm, relaxed voice as you summarize the situation as you see it. You could say something like, "Your mother needs to make a decision about where to go for rehabilitation. Let's go discuss with your mother the advantages and disadvantages of each of the places that are suited to meet her needs. She needs support from both of you on whatever she decides."

The assertive Leveler makes honest statements that are direct and to the point. His posture is relaxed and open. He maintains direct eye contact but doesn't stare, and hand gestures and body movements are slow and relaxed. An assertive Leveler can control his temper when people get angry and start to yell. He asks questions to understand and analyze a situation. He speaks up and asks clearly for what he wants, and can say no to requests without feeling guilty.

Do you know anyone who could fit any of these descriptions? Do you see yourself in any of them? Some of you are bound in these patterns of behavior because you've used them for years to deal with stress and anxiety. As a professional nurse, however, you must learn to become more of a Leveler. One way to start is by carefully analyzing situations that you find stressful and irritating. What upset you? How did you react? What did you want from yourself? What did you want from the other person? Learning to manage stressful situations by leveling is very important, and will be covered in depth in Chapter 5.

SUMMARY

Therapeutic communication is used to establish and maintain collaborative relationships with patients. In contrast, failure to use therapeutic communication techniques will result in stress for both you and your patients. It will also cause conflict in the relationship. Not every patient relationship results in the attainment of health goals and objectives. However, the more skilled at therapeutic communication you become, the better you'll be able to establish trusting collaborative relationships that will maximize the chance of efficiently and effectively accomplishing mutual goals and objectives. In addition, patient and family satisfaction will be high. Your patients will be exclaiming how wonderful the care was and how well they were treated.

Remember that communication is both verbal and nonverbal. Body language, appearance, and tone of voice are more significant than the actual words you speak as you attempt to deliver a message. Remembering the following four basic principles of therapeutic communication will help you send and interpret messages as accurately as possible.

- Verify that a message has been received correctly by paying careful attention to feedback.
- Carefully size up your patient's nonverbal cues, including body language and facial expressions. Also, become conscious of your own nonverbal cues.
- Personal appearance—such as hygiene, grooming, and clothing—make a loud statement that can facilitate or hinder communication.
- When nonverbal behavior and tone of voice don't match a person's spoken words, respond to the nonverbal message and tone of voice, not the spoken words.

No one can attain perfect therapeutic communication or perfect communication of any form. You can't read the minds and hearts of those with whom you communicate, and they can't read yours, so you'll probably misinterpret some aspect of a message from time to time. Patients will misinterpret you as well, especially when they're anxious or afraid. However, you can and should continually strive to improve your ability to accurately grasp the main points of a message and send appropriate messages in return. In some situations, this is much easier said than done.

COMMUNICATE?

If we have difficulty understanding or being understood, it is likely we have ignored some part of the communication process. It is up to us, individually, to try to find the problem and correct it.

The following self-evaluation can help you assess your particular areas of need and interest and provide you with a standard by which you can measure your progress. Circle the number that best represents the frequency of each item in your experience.

Seldom
  Sometimes
    Often
      Usually

1	2	3	4	**a)**	People understand my thoughts and feelings.
1	2	3	4	**b)**	When communication problems arise, I am determined to solve them.
1	2	3	4	**c)**	I know the major causes of communication breakdown.
1	2	3	4	**d)**	I demonstrate personality qualities to which people are attracted.
1	2	3	4	**e)**	In difficult situations, I consciously choose how I express myself.
1	2	3	4	**f)**	The tone of my voice and the words I say communicate precisely how I feel about my conversational partner.
1	2	3	4	**g)**	I am able to listen deeply to the feelings expressed by my spouse and friends.
1	2	3	4	**h)**	My friends tell me I am a good listener.
1	2	3	4	**i)**	I can tell whether a communication problem is basically caused by the one speaking, the message itself, or the listener to the message.
1	2	3	4	**j)**	I am able to analyze accurately the thoughts and feelings of the person talking to me.
1	2	3	4	**k)**	When I talk, people listen.
1	2	3	4	**l)**	People tell me I am a good conversationalist.
1	2	3	4	**m)**	I say no when I want to say no.
1	2	3	4	**n)**	I assert myself because I value my own opinions as well as the opinion of others.
1	2	3	4	**o)**	I handle hassles with children effectively.

Seldom
  Sometimes
    Often
      Usually

HOW WELL DO YOU COMMUNICATE? *(continued)*

1 2 3 4	**p)**	I talk with children the way I want them to talk to me.
1 2 3 4	**q)**	I allow loved ones and friends to know me as I really am.
1 2 3 4	**r)**	I am able to tell people close to me how much I really care about them.
1 2 3 4	**s)**	When I experience a conflict with someone, I know how to resolve it.
1 2 3 4	**t)**	I know what to say in tense situations.
1 2 3 4	**u)**	I know how to gain the cooperation of others.
1 2 3 4	**v)**	When I ask people to do something that I want them to do (within reason), they do it.
1 2 3 4	**w)**	I enjoy the highest level of communication with family, friends, and business associates.
1 2 3 4	**x)**	Because I know the value of successful communication, I look for ways to improve my communication skills.

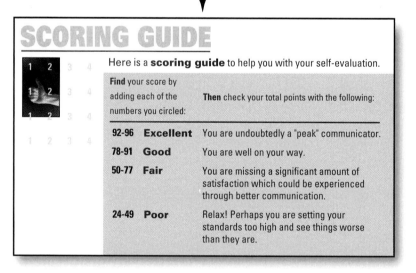

SCORING GUIDE

Here is a **scoring guide** to help you with your self-evaluation.

Find your score by adding each of the numbers you circled: **Then** check your total points with the following:

92-96	**Excellent**	You are undoubtedly a "peak" communicator.
78-91	**Good**	You are well on your way.
50-77	**Fair**	You are missing a significant amount of satisfaction which could be experienced through better communication.
24-49	**Poor**	Relax! Perhaps you are setting your standards too high and see things worse than they are.

Swets, P: The Art of Talking So That People Will Listen. Simon and Schuster, New York, 1983. Adapted and reprinted with permission.

COMMUNICATION EXERCISES

1. On pages 25–26 is a communication assessment to help you identify your own areas of need related to the general communication process.[11] If you get a high score, good for you! If you don't do as well as you would have liked, however, don't despair. You can learn to be a good communicator, and you can learn to use therapeutic communication techniques. You'll find out much more about them in later chapters.

2. Recall a difficult communication you had recently. It doesn't have to be with a patient. It could be with a family member, a friend, a student, or a coworker. Think about the setting, the circumstances surrounding the conflict, and the reactions (verbal and nonverbal) of those involved. Now make a two-column table. In the first column, record your verbal and nonverbal messages. In the second column, record the other person's verbal and nonverbal messages. What got you upset? With which communication style did you react? What did you want for yourself? What did you want from the other person? What could you have done to respond more like a Leveler?

3. Use the outcomes of the nursing communications diagram on page 8 and the Life Fields Communication Theory on page 15 to analyze the difficult communication described in exercise 2.

References

1. National Organization of Nurse Practitioner Faculties: Advanced Nursing Practice: Curriculum Guidelines and Program Standards for Nurse Practitioner Education. National Organization of Nurse Practitioner Faculties, Washington, D.C., 1995.
2. Shannon, C, and Weaver, E: The Mathematical Theory of Communication. University of Illinois Press, Champaign, Illinois, 1949.
3. Leary, T: The theory and measurement methodology of interpersonal communication. Psychiatry 18:147, 1955.
4. Mehrabian, A: Nonverbal Communication. Aldine-Atherton, Inc, Chicago, Illinois, 1972.
5. Mehrabian, A, and Williams, M: Nonverbal concomitants of perceived and intended persuasiveness. Journal of Personality and Social Psychology 13(1):37, 1969.

6. Combs, AW, Avila, DL, and Purkey, WW: The Helping Relationship Sourcebook. Allyn & Bacon, Boston, 1971.
7. Grimes, J, and Burns, E: Health Assessment in Nursing Practice. Little Brown Company, Boston, Massachusetts, 1996.
8. Selye, H: The Stress of Life. McGraw-Hill, New York, 1976.
9. Maslow, A: Motivation and Personality. Harper & Row, New York, 1970.
10. Potter, PA, and Perry, AG: Fundamentals of Nursing: Concepts, Process, and Practice, ed 4. Mosby, St. Louis, 1997.
11. Satir, V: Conjoint Family Therapy. Science and Behavior Books, Palo Alto, California, 1964.
12. Satir, V. The New Peoplemaking. Science and Behavior Books, Mountain View, California, 1988.
13. Swets, P. The Art of Talking So That People Will Listen: Getting Through to Family, Friends, and Business Associates. Simon and Schuster, New York, 1983.

Suggested Further Reading

Elgin, SH: The Gentle Art of Verbal Self-Defense. Dorset Press, New York, 1980. (Learn how to detect and respond to typical verbal "put-downs").

Gender Differences in Communication

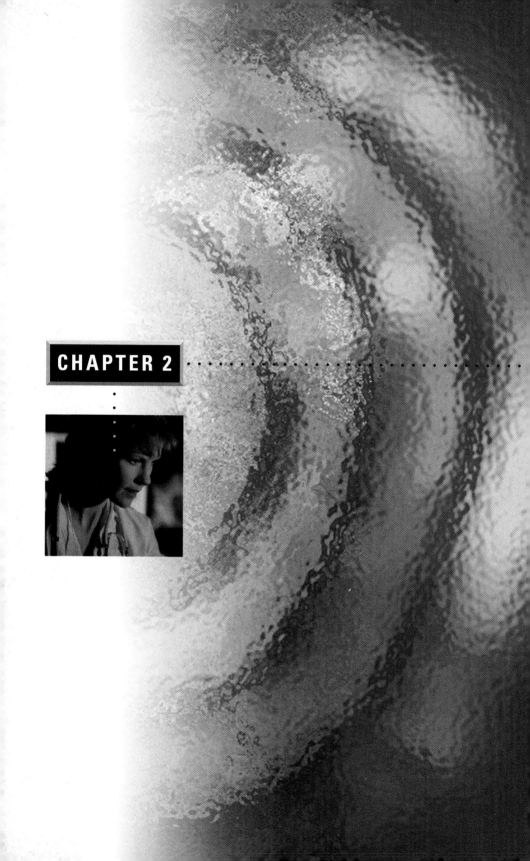

CHAPTER 2

Gender Differences in Communication

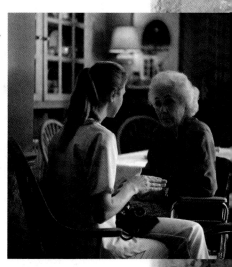

Chapter Objectives

AFTER READING THIS CHAPTER,
YOU WILL BE ABLE TO:

1. Identify the importance of understanding gender differences in communication.
2. Explain the influence of culture on gender communication.
3. Describe biologically based gender differences in communication.
4. Describe the typical purpose and styles of communication for men and women.
5. Apply the principles of gender differences in communication with patients and other healthcare professionals.
6. Describe gender differences related to the communication of discomfort.

THE FOCUS OF THIS CHAPTER IS ON GENDER DIFFERENCES IN COMMUNICA-tion. As you communicate with patients or other healthcare providers, you need to recognize typical gender-based language patterns to send and interpret messages more clearly. Once you recognize and understand gender-based language patterns, you'll be better able to understand the perspective of the other person and to alter your communication patterns to establish therapeutic or collaborative relationships.

The major theoretical basis for this chapter is from research in the field of social linguistics. The cartoon on page 32 illustrates stereotyp-ical gender differences in communication. Typically, women's speech has been stereotyped as stupid, vague, emotional, confused, and wordy in communication patterns, whereas men's speech has been stereotyped as logical, concise, businesslike, and controlled in com-

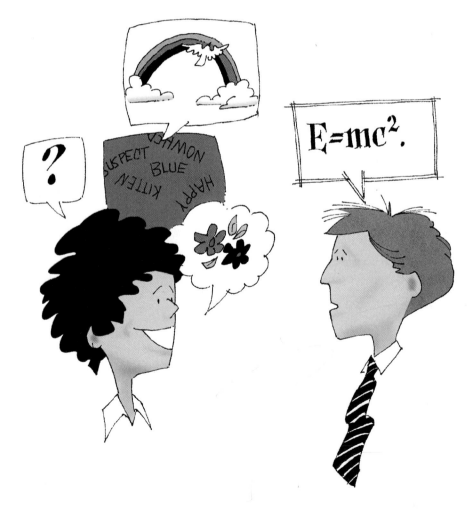

munication.[1] However, these stereotypes don't indicate the real differences based on evidence from scientific research.[1-3]

To communicate effectively with other professionals and therapeutically with patients, you must learn to recognize and understand gender differences. Also, you must be able to take each person's language style into account, adjusting your style of communication when you detect differences in communication styles based on culturally derived assumptions and values about gender.

Identifying Patterns of Verbal and Nonverbal Communication

We all recognize that each person is a unique individual, but we also tend to see others as representatives of groups. It's a natural tendency to see patterns in the world and to group things in our minds according to these categories. Grouping items into categories is useful because it helps predict behaviors. However, placing individual human beings into categories is offensive to many people. Human beings are unique, shaped by religion, ethnic background, race, age, profession, social class, regions of the country and world that they've visited and lived in, as well as numerous other life experiences and personality factors.

If you make broad generalizations, individual differences become obscured and you may be accused of stereotyping. Stereotyping occurs when a person makes a conclusion about someone else based on a broad category. Examples of stereotypes are the stubborn German, southern belle, hot-blooded Italian, New York Jew, Texas cowboy, and so on. These categories might be useful in predicting some behavior, but they miss a lot more than they predict. They're also misleading and usually insulting to the person placed in the category.

Regarding gender differences, stereotypes that you have probably heard before include the dumb blonde or aggressive man. Remember that anyone placed in a stereotypical cultural or gender category remains unique, different from everyone else, including other people who might be placed in the same category.

The idea that women and men are different may lead to the conclusion that the difference justifies unequal treatment and unequal opportunity. Women may fear that observations of gender differences may imply that women are different from the "normal" standard of whatever men are, making them inferior to men. Likewise, a statement such as, "You men are all alike," coming from a woman to a man, may be interpreted as an accusation that objectifies and slanders him.

However, real differences do exist in the way in which men and women communicate, much of which is culturally derived. These differences in style are based on research by sociolinguistic researchers such as Deborah Tannen.[2] She suggests that "the risk of ignoring differences between men and women is much greater than the danger of naming them" (p. 16). The purpose of recognizing gender differences in styles of communication is to understand ourselves and members of the opposite sex, and to apply this knowledge to facilitate communication between men and women.

CULTURAL INFLUENCES ON GENDER COMMUNICATIONS

Gender differences in communication have been referred to as cross-cultural communication; they reflect differences in the beliefs and practices of men and women in the way in which they relate to their worlds. Many cultural factors influence the way in which men and women communicate. Cultural beliefs involve the ideas and practices passed down through the ages. You have developed beliefs throughout your life about which types of verbal and nonverbal behaviors are acceptable for men and women. Cultural beliefs are translated into social behaviors and communication patterns that are taught and transmitted by your family and religion, and they are affected by the prevailing culture of the society in which you live.

You need to recognize the cultural influences within yourself as you communicate with patients, and you need to identify the cultural influences affecting how patients communicate. The focus of this chapter is on gender and communication. Keep in mind, however, that there are many other cultural differences between people in addition to the way they communicate. Each of us needs to get beyond the census data that classifies us as Asian, African American, Caucasian, Native American, Hispanic, and others. This classification lends itself to stereotyping and the assumption that all members of a group are alike.

There are multiple groups of people within each classification, each group with differing belief systems and ways of practicing those beliefs. You may be able to identify your ethnic roots and, if asked, would report being Italian, Jewish, German, Polish, Swedish, English, African, Japanese, or some combination. If you are a citizen of the United States or Canada, you probably consider yourself American or Canadian. However, only Native Americans can claim to be fully American. The rest of us had ancestors who came here by either boat or plane. Those ancestors brought a culture with them that has been passed down to us. We have all been affected by ethnic backgrounds, but some of us may be more aware of it than others.

The brief cultural assessment on page 35 will help you become aware of your own cultural values, attitudes, and practices and how these affect your communication with patients and families. For ex-

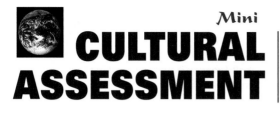

Mini
CULTURAL ASSESSMENT

Please assess yourself, then we'll exchange views with others from the same and different ethnic backgrounds

▶ **To what culture/ethnic group do you belong?**

▶ **In what country were you born?**

▶ **In what country were parents or grandparents (ancestors) born?**

▶ **How closely do you associate with your ethnic group?**

▶ **Whom do you consider your family?**

▶ **How important to you is your family?**

▶ **In your family, who takes care of infants and children?**

▶ In your family, who takes care of sick or elderly?

▶ What do you believe about marriage?

▶ What do you believe about childbearing?

▶ How do you view a nursing mother?

▶ Do you think you should try to control the environment or live in harmony with it?

▶ What is the meaning of life?

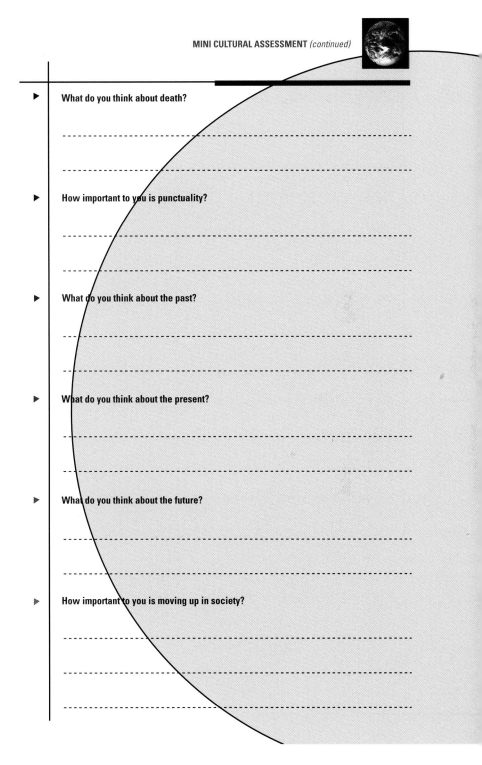

▶ **What do you think about death?**

_____

_____

▶ **How important to you is punctuality?**

_____

_____

▶ **What do you think about the past?**

_____

_____

▶ **What do you think about the present?**

_____

_____

▶ **What do you think about the future?**

_____

_____

▶ **How important to you is moving up in society?**

_____

_____

_____

▶ **What are the traditional roles of family members in your culture?**

▶ **Who does what tasks in your family?**

▶ **How are decisions made in your family?**

▶ **What place do elderly relatives have in your life?**

▶ **Is the sex of a baby important? Are girl and boy infants treated differently?**

▶ **What rules govern sexual activity for a man? For a woman?**

----

ample, were boys and girls treated differently in the family in which you grew up? In some families with Italian ethnic customs, the women wait on the men and take care of the children and the sick, men usually head the household, and the religious upbringing is typically Roman Catholic. Italians are typically expressive of their thoughts and emotions. When a family member is sick, the extended family—including aunts, uncles, and cousins—typically gathers around.

There are many ramifications from the culture that affect communication in nursing. For example, a patient's response to pain may range from stoicism to crying, screaming, and writhing.[4] If your background taught you to value self-control, you must not impose your values on the patient. Instead, you need to view the way in which a patient's response to pain is communicated within the cultural context. Your nursing goal is to recognize verbal and nonverbal pain responses, and to intervene to alleviate discomfort.

Communication patterns are culturally ingrained into gender roles. A gender role consists of different activities that men and women engage in with different frequencies. The concept of "role" can be traced back to terminology used in the theater. The role was the paper the script was written on. Thus, male and female gender roles are the scripts that men and women follow to fulfill their parts in acting masculine or feminine.[3] The roles of women and men are culturally encouraged patterns of behavior. Thus, verbal and nonverbal behaviors for communication are part of gender role scripts.

Examples of gender roles relevant to communication include the gender behaviors of women as gentle and emotional, compared with the gender behavior of men as powerful and in control of their feelings. Are all women gentle and all men not gentle? Are all men powerful and all women not powerful? Are all men in control of their feelings at all times, and are all women emotional? Of course not! As soon as you say all men or all women, you are stereotyping people. You can, however, identify role communication patterns that are more typically prevalent in one gender over the other. In this case, you are not stereotyping. You are classifying and identifying typical behavior patterns pertinent to communication based on gender.

Gender roles with resulting verbal and nonverbal styles have changed over time because of the changing needs of our society. Our ideas about acceptable gender-specific behaviors in others and ourselves are constantly under revision. For example, at one time, predominant gender roles had men as breadwinners and women as homemakers. This is not true any longer. Many women now work outside the home.

You need to evaluate the basis for the gender differences in communication and recognize cultural gender role differences in communication. Once these differences are known, you can change your communication patterns to become better able to communicate with patients and also become better at professional communication with other healthcare providers.

BIOLOGICAL INFLUENCES ON GENDER COMMUNICATION

Although brain research is still in its infancy, neurologists suggest that there are structural and chemical differences in the brains of men and women.[3,5,6] The brain and spinal cord are anatomically and neuro-chemically complex, with more than 50 billion neurons in the cerebral hemispheres alone.[7] Brain research has been stymied because animal brains are inadequate to represent a model of the human brain for testing, and it is ethically and morally obvious that scientists cannot experiment with human brains in the same way they do with animal brains. Thus, relatively little is known about the human brain compared with the anatomy and physiology of other tissues of the human body.

However, research to date indicates that female brains are less lateralized during speech. Women use both sides of the brain, whereas men use primarily the left side of the brain, regardless of whether they are right-handed or left-handed.[6] In addition, men's brains are under the influence of the hormone testosterone, whereas women's brains are primarily under the influence of the hormones estrogen and pro-gesterone.[3,5,7] These hormones are important to sexual development and behavior.

Hormones also affect behavior. For example, male bodies produce 10 to 40 times more testosterone than female bodies do.[7] Research suggests that aggressive behaviors may be linked to hormonal abnor-malities, and that men with higher-than-average testosterone levels exhibit a wide variety of antisocial behaviors.[3] Among women, pre-menstrual syndrome (PMS) is a neuroendocrine disorder that causes depression, anger, irritability, tension, fatigue, and confusion.[7] It is be-lieved that mood changes in PMS may result from altered serotonin transmission in the central nervous system. Selective serotonin re-uptake inhibitors are considered the drug of choice to treat PMS. It is interesting to note that hormone levels are the same in women who experience PMS and those who do not. However, it has been hypothe-sized that those with PMS may be more sensitive to hormonal changes.[7]

It will take many more years to sort out the biological and cultural differences in communication. In the meantime, researchers agree that men and women have different styles of speech.[1-3] Your personal experiences communicating with members of the opposite sex may have already led you to the conclusion that differences do exist in communication patterns, although you may not have recognized and classified the differences in styles of speech.

Styles of Speech

Tannen's research identified several differences in the styles of speech between men and women (primarily North American).[2] In her book, she compares and contrasts gender differences that may become barriers during communication.

Tannen's research suggests that the communication style of women typically focuses on intimacy and forming communal connections, whereas many men have a style of communication that focuses on hierarchy and the attaining and demonstration of status. Gray has characterized the gender differences in styles communication as worlds apart, and wrote a popular book entitled *Men are from Mars, Women are from Venus*.[8] The title is, of course, a humorous overstatement, but there is resounding agreement between researchers that gender differences do exist in styles of communication.

RAPPORT TALK VERSUS REPORT TALK

Tannen suggests that communication tends to be unbalanced because men and women talk to accomplish different purposes.[2] According to Tannen, for most women, the preferred language of everyday conversation is that of rapport. Women are interested in establishing and negotiating intimate, sympathetic, harmonious relationships. They want to establish connection, display similarities, and match experiences. The essence of female friendship is to get together to talk about what they think and feel about a situation, with careful attention to details of what happened and who was there. It is important to them to share thoughts and impressions. Women will call each other on the phone just to "chat" and ask in general about how things are going and make "small talk." Many women are most comfortable having private conversations, perhaps because of the intimate, personal nature of the content of their messages. As a result, many women can express what they are feeling better than many men can.

Rapport talk needs to be differentiated from destructive gossip, however. The difference between rapport talk (small talk), often characteristic of women, and gossip, is the purpose of the type of talk. The stereotype of "gossiping women" has a negative connotation. The most negative connotation of gossip is that it is destructive and involves rumors, slander, and defamation of character. Gossip does not create rapport between individuals. It destroys relationships.

In contrast, the purpose of small talk for many women is to develop rapport and to facilitate relationships. If you realize that many women make small talk to establish rapport, even if you personally prefer a more direct or technical approach to a conversation, you become better able to understand the purpose of the other person's conversational style. In addition, it is interesting to note that, in terms of total talking time observed in conversations, men spend more time talking than women.[1]

Characteristic of male language is report talk. Men generally prefer a style of language that involves freely announcing and stating facts to give an account, with a "skip-the-details" approach. Even the most private situations can be approached as though giving a report. Men are typically great debaters—direct and straightforward in speech. They are often more comfortable than women when talking in large groups that may be made up of people they do not know well.

In contrast to the speech style of many women, who seek to develop harmonious relationships through rapport speech, the purpose of the report style of speech for many men is to assert independence and to maintain or augment status in social groups. Tannen suggests that many men like to be the ones to impart information and appear knowledgeable about a topic and give advice.

The focus of many men on being independent and having status may translate into a style of conversation that centers on a preference for telling others what to do. Telling others what to do increases independence and status, whereas taking orders lowers status and decreases independence. Many men like to exhibit knowledge and skill, holding center stage through verbal performance to demonstrate independence and status. For example, many men like to tell success stories about their accomplishments.

Tannen gives many examples of imbalances between men telling stories about their accomplishments and women listening without interrupting. Later, however, the women may report being very bored and not enjoying the conversation because it was so one-sided and out of balance with the exchange of ideas and information. If everyone takes turns talking and listening, more participants report satisfaction with the conversation.

Rapport and Reporting Skills for Nurses

Regardless of the healthcare setting in which you work, you will spend much of your time talking to patients and family members, other nurses, and other members of the healthcare team. Rapport talk with patients is essential to therapeutic communication because rapport talk leads to the development of trusting therapeutic relationships. Nurses typically take a patient-centered approach focused on interpersonal relationships with patients and their significant others.[9] Nurses also tend to focus on developing sympathetic and harmonious relationships.

To care for patients successfully, you'll need to assess carefully their physical and emotional responses and their adjustment to the hospital, clinic, or home care setting. You'll learn the most intimate details of the patient's health status and family situation, and then apply your knowledge as a health professional to provide physical and emotional support, guidance, and teaching.

For example, you will routinely assess urinary and bowel elimination. If a patient has a problem, you may catheterize the bladder or administer an enema. You'll need to pay close attention to the patient's emotional response, use anticipatory guidance, and give lots of encouragement throughout the procedure. You may have to teach a patient how to catheterize herself or administer her own enema. If you have developed a therapeutic relationship and rapport before performing the procedure, and then continue to build rapport during the procedure, your patient will be more apt to trust you, cooperate with you, and be satisfied with the care you gave.

You will routinely use a therapeutic communication skill called distraction. Distraction involves the use of small talk, and thus serves to build harmonious relationships. For this technique, you simply engage a patient in conversation to take her mind off a problem. For example, while giving a patient a bath, you'd want to put the person at ease because of the intimacy of the procedure. Engaging a patient in rapport talk may be helpful. For example, if pictures, cards, or flowers are in the room, ask about them as a way of getting into a conversation. Sharing some information about yourself is another way of getting into a conversation to develop rapport. For example, "Those pictures of your children are great. I have four children." The point isn't to talk about your own children, of course. It's to encourage the patient to talk about her own family and to establish rapport while distracting the patient from the procedure.

Some patients may prefer report talk as a means to distract them therapeutically. If the patient is reading a newspaper or watching the news, try engaging the patient in conversation by asking a general question, such as, "Is anything interesting going on in the news today?" Then encourage the patient to tell you all about their favorite news and opinions of what is happening in the news. This will likely distract him from the intimacy of a procedure such as a bed bath.

You also need to know how to report information and whom to ask for information with a "skip-the-details" approach. For example, when you give an end-of-shift report to other nurses, you'll want to provide only critical information. If you work in a public health or community setting, you'll be calling other healthcare providers to give reports or ask for information about patients in your care. In talking with physicians about patients, report talk is definitely indicated. Physicians focus on the pathophysiology and are interested in a brief summary of the patient's physiological status. So tell the physician about vital signs and head-to-toe assessment data specific to the patient's malfunctioning physiological systems. Especially if you're getting a physician out of bed to give a report at 3 AM, make sure you have the physiological status report in order. Skip the interpersonal relationships and emotional responses; the physician's aim is to fix the pathology with medications and surgery. He'll be interested in information specific to his focus on pathology.

You must know the correct information to report to each healthcare worker, and you must learn when to make referrals to other healthcare providers. For example, you'll need to know specifically which assessment data to report to the dietitian, the physical therapist, the respiratory therapist, and the social worker, in addition to knowing what to report and refer to the physician.

Status and Power in Relationships

Physicians, whether male or female, are independent and have high social status. Typically, the doctor asks the questions, the patient gives the answers, and then the doctor gives advice. Physicians write "orders" for patients, and nurses carry out the orders. Nurses also get on the phone and talk to physicians when something is going wrong with the patient to get an "order." This may be why nurses are stereotyped as doing the bidding of others. The cartoon on page 45 depicts stereotypical physician-nurse communication.

Nurses are given little public credit for their ability to make decisions, nor are they awarded recognition for their contribution to patient care. In reality, nurses carefully check orders and question any order that does not make sense. Some physicians are grateful. A few may interpret the questions as an attack on their ability to practice medicine. But it is your responsibility to help and not harm your patients. So you shouldn't follow a physician's orders blindly. If an order doesn't make sense to you, you must assume responsibility for questioning the order.

If you talk to a physician about an order and you still believe it to be wrong after the discussion, you have the right to refuse to carry out the order based on your belief that it will harm your patient or jeopar-

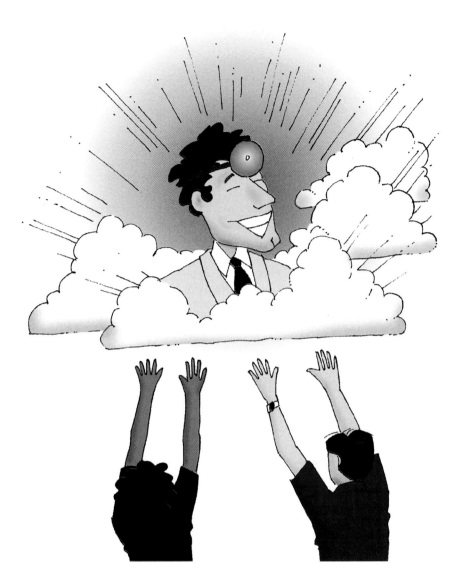

dize his safety. You should discuss this problem with your nursing supervisor, who may need to assist you in managing the situation. A
strong clinical knowledge base combined with excellent assessment
and communication skills will help you successfully protect and defend the safety of your patients. In addition, your clinical knowledge
and communication skills form the basis of your power in relationships with other healthcare providers.

LESS ADVERSATIVE VERSUS MORE ADVERSATIVE

The word adversative is defined as pitting one's own needs, wants, and skills against those of others. In this context, it involves conflict, and it is an essential part of human nature. The way you learn to manage conflict may be related to the types of games you played as a child. Janet Lever studied fifth graders at play.[10] Boys' games involved complex rules and roles and relied on skills. In contrast, girls' games involved complexity in verbally managing interpersonal relations. Girls' games were contests but not of skill. Rather, games became a popularity contest. Lever suggested that the social games children play as they grow up contribute to the formation of adult responses to conflict.

To many women, conflict is a threat to connection and should be avoided. The goal of conversation for many women is to strive for peace and harmony. Women usually prefer to settle disputes without direct confrontation. Some women avoid confrontation at all cost, and are virtually incapable of expressing anger and conflict. When it comes to a career and the workplace, women often place higher value on affiliation and collective goals than on personal achievement. Women are inclined to sacrifice personal needs for the needs of the group. When it comes to making decisions, women tend to take into account more factors, with a higher sensitivity to personal and moral aspects of a problem.[2]

Many men are much more comfortable with competition and conflict. If the conflict is friendly, it becomes a means of bonding. Friendship involves competition and friendly aggression. For example, many men thrive on football or other sports. If they don't participate in the sport themselves, they have a favorite team to support. Many men enjoy the socially acceptable violence and aggression of a sport. In other examples, men typically compete to be the best golfer in the place where they work, or they may tell stories about catching the biggest fish. This carries over into the professional workplace, where men aggressively compete to meet their professional goals and thrive on beating others out of the top spot.

The perspective of many men is that some people are on top and some are on the bottom when it comes to status in a social group. To many men, this is a part of life. Everyone has a function and everyone is not equal. Men typically are not as interested in popularity as women are. Men may be more interested in being respected by others than in being liked by others. Of course, everyone wants to be liked. But to many men, if it comes down to a choice between being liked or respected, they would probably prefer to be respected.

Nurses and Adversity

As a nurse, whether you are male or female, you must learn to manage conflict. You may encounter conflicts over scheduling or patient assignments, appropriate treatment measures, ethical issues, and other differences, regardless of the setting in which you work. If you have trouble dealing with adversity and conflict, you'll need to come to terms with that problem. For example, if you identify a problem or a solution to a problem, you need to be able to speak out and be direct about what's wrong and how the problem could be resolved. Although diplomacy and tact are essential skills, too much politeness may dilute the message.

You also must develop sensitivity to the moral and social aspects of patient care situations by learning to become a patient advocate. Advocacy in nursing means that you must speak up to defend human rights—the right of patients to make their own decisions, for example. Developing strategies for communication during conflict will be discussed further in Chapter 5.

COOPERATIVE OVERLAPPING VERSUS TALKING ALONE

In a communication pattern known as overlapping, a listener may talk along with the speaker, yet the speaker isn't annoyed or disturbed by the intrusion. The purpose of the overlap is to show support, interest, cooperation, and emotional ties. In contrast, an interruption is considered to be a violation of speaking rights and, thus, to be inconsiderate.

Whether or not a speaker considers the person talking with him or her to be overlapping or interrupting depends partly on culture. For example, many Italians, Asians, and Filipinos value talking together. Most North Americans believe that one person should speak at a time, although North American women overlap more than men do in an attempt to build relationships. In many cases, North American men may consider the overlap an interruption, especially if they prefer to hold center stage as a means to demonstrate independence and status.

Actually, men and women often complain that each interrupts the other. Many women say that their messages are often interrupted with, "Get to the point." On the other hand, many men may consider an overlap as an interruption, although the person may have been trying to show support with the overlap. Those who believe that they should talk alone, regardless of gender, consider an overlap to be rude. Research indicates that men interrupt women considerably more often than women interrupt men.[11]

The key to whether overlap becomes an interruption depends on whether or not the conversation is balanced. If one speaker repeatedly overlaps and the other gives way, the conversation is unbalanced and the effect is one of domination and interruption. If both speakers cooperatively overlap each other and neither gives way for the other, there is balance and harmony.

Nurses and Interruption

To communicate therapeutically, you need to aim for a balanced conversation. If the patient overlaps you in conversation, then you can overlap too. If the patient does not overlap you as you speak, then let him speak alone and don't overlap. You'll need to develop the sensitivity to discern a patient's preferences for overlapping or speaking alone.

If you feel that you're being interrupted, you must learn to speak up and say, "Please let me finish what I was saying" or "Please let me finish first." On the other hand, if you're in the habit of interrupting, take a deep breath, hold it a second, and really listen to what the other person is trying to say as you exhale.

LISTENER VERSUS INFORMATION PROVIDER

Many women typically listen more, whereas many men typically seek opportunities to give information. Again, this pattern may reflect the female attempt to build relationships with active listening, playing down expertise rather than displaying it to promote harmony. In contrast, men may value the center stage while speaking because it gives them the feeling of knowing more and having importance and status. With one person talking and the other person listening, an unbalanced relationship occurs, with the giver of information having a higher status than the listener.

When men speak to each other, they may try to challenge the content of the message, match information given with their own expertise in the area, or sidetrack the speaker to a different topic. Men may view these behaviors as an exchange of information between two equals. Many men may have the impression that people who do not challenge or match information with their own expertise do not know anything about the topic and therefore do not join in the conversation. Some men may feel obliged to keep on lecturing. In contrast, many women may view challenges and sidetracks as rude, nonlistening behaviors that will break down relationships (although they may be bored listening to a lecture). Thus, women and men may be mutually dissatisfied with the arrangement of women typically listening and men typically providing information.

Many women are more inclined to give listening responses, murmuring "Yes" as encouragement for the speaker to continue, and nodding the head to provide feedback and encourage a relationship. In contrast, men typically focus on the message and its literal meanings, and will say what they mean in return. Therefore, men say "yes" and nod only if they agree. Women also tend to ask more questions to encourage further verbal expressions, whereas men do not. Women may attempt to draw quieter members of a group into a conversation, whereas men may assume that anyone who has something to say will volunteer it.[12]

Sometimes people may give the impression they are not listening even when they are, simply because of differences in communication styles. Many men tend to avoid eye contact because it makes them feel uncomfortable. If a person expects feedback from a listener, however, it becomes frustrating to talk to someone who sits silently and avoids eye contact. When the purpose of speech is to express intimacy, it also may frustrate the speaker if the listener makes statements rather than asking questions and issues challenges rather than agreeing with the speaker. If the speaker is hoping and expecting to receive verbal and nonverbal support from the listener and instead becomes frustrated, the relationship will deteriorate.

It's also important to recognize that some people, regardless of gender, really don't want to listen to someone else at length because they feel that listening makes them subordinate and that the person talking is dominant over them. The act of giving information is of higher status than listening. It is noteworthy that, although a person may be an unwilling listener, he will listen quietly to a lecture from a supervisor because the supervisor has a higher status.

A strategy of women who need to establish professional relationships with men may be to listen politely and show interest even though they're not at all interested. The woman may be focused on the interdependence of relationships and the promotion of harmony. In contrast, men may attempt to offer interesting information to establish professional relationships with women. The difference in style is the result of habit and differing goals of asserting individuality and status versus a focus on harmony during interpersonal relationships.

Nurses and Listening versus Providing Information

To be therapeutic, you must learn to listen actively and also to provide information. Listening is a crucial skill. Listening responses—such as nodding your head or saying "Yes" or "Go on" as a patient speaks—are an effective means of showing a patient that you're interested and that you want her to continue talking. Effective listening skills will be fully described in Chapter 5.

In contrast, if you find yourself talking a lot and the patient doing all the listening, the conversation is out of balance. Stop talking and ask a question of the patient to draw him into the conversation. Ask the patient for his ideas or opinions. You may even ask a question to determine whether the patient is following what you're trying to say or teach. Otherwise, the person may be just listening politely, either not really interested in what you're saying or not really understanding you. By stopping yourself from talking, you also give the other person an opportunity to change the topic to something that is of interest to him.

STORYTELLING

Most people, regardless of gender, like to tell stories. Storytelling involves exchanging accounts of personal experiences. The stories that women tell tend to revolve around relationships. For example, women may like to talk about how they met their mates. Stories often center on the violation of social norms of the community and joint actions by groups. Women prefer to tell stories of peculiar people and dramatize abnormal behavior.

Men typically like to tell stories of human contests. They tell stories of how they acted alone and report a happy outcome in an adventure in which they come out on top. Rarely do they receive help or advice from someone else. For example, they may describe contests with nature involving hunting and fishing.

Nurses, Patients, and Storytelling

By listening to patients' stories, you can help distract them from their problems, as described earlier in the chapter. Other therapeutic communication interventions involving storytelling include reminiscence and life review, in which the patient recalls and talks about her past life experiences. Reminiscing can be helpful in resocializing people and building relationships, and a life review can help a person make sense of her life and see it as a unique story. You can implement reminiscence or life reviews to help patients deal with crises and losses, to prevent and reduce depression, and to increase life satisfaction.[13]

Nurses also like to tell stories. However, you must be very careful to avoid telling stories about patients, because it may be considered a breech of patient confidentiality. Naturally, you need to talk about patients with other healthcare providers to develop, implement, and evaluate the plan of care. However, patient confidentiality requires that you not mention patient names outside the patient care setting or discuss confidential information with anyone not directly involved in the patient's care. This includes not talking about patients in hospital elevators, cafeterias, corridors, or any place where the conversation could be overheard.

When family members or friends inquire about a patient's diagnosis or prognosis, tell them to discuss these confidential matters directly with the patient or the physician. If the patient's family or friends ask a general question about how the patient is doing today, it's fine to give a general answer. However, the specifics of the diagnosis and prognosis are strictly confidential.

Gender Differences in Language Use

In addition to the gender differences discussed so far, men and women may show varying patterns when it comes to specific language usage, as in tag questions and conversational rituals.

TAG QUESTIONS

Some women tend to ask more questions than men, commonly in the form of tag questions. In this type of language usage, the speaker adds a phrase at the end of a statement that turns it into a question: "I'd like to go out to eat - wouldn't you?" Women may use this form to hear the other's thoughts on the subject and encourage the expression of opinions. However, if the woman really wants to go out to dinner, she'd be better off making a statement, such as, "I'd like to go out to dinner tonight."

The danger of tag questions is that the other person, especially a man, not aware of the purpose of the tag question, may answer with a personal opinion such as "I'd rather stay in tonight." If he had known that the speaker really wanted to go out, he might have gone along happily. Men are sometimes prone to respond more literally to questions and, therefore, may misinterpret some forms of questions. A man may simply give an honest answer, but he may get in trouble because the woman asking the question may interpret his answer to mean, "I don't like you because I don't want to go out even when I know you do."

Another phrase used as a tag is, "What do you think?" The purpose is to make others feel involved and ask for other opinions before making a decision. Women aim to make decisions by consensus. However, a problem occurs if the person to whom the tag question was directed interprets this to mean, "Make the decision for me." The tag question has given the impression that the speaker lacks the confidence to make the decision.

Many women also ask "Why" questions more often than men ask them. They seek an explanation, perhaps in an attempt to understand the other's thoughts on the subject. The net effect of tag questions during conversations is that women may appear less intelligent or uncertain.

Nursing and Tag Questions

Your ability to ask questions is very important in allowing you to develop a better understanding of a situation and to devise solutions to problems. It's important to solicit the input of everyone involved in a situation before carefully analyzing data to make a better decision. However, tag questions typically aren't useful.

Instead of a tag, make a direct and polite statement about what you would like to be done. For example, in a nursing home, a statement and tag question can get you into trouble. "It's time for your bath, don't you think?" may result in the patient saying, "No, I think I want to skip it today." If you really want something to get done right away because of the schedule, don't ask a question, make a statement. Don't give a person a choice if there really isn't one. If you make a statement, the patient still has the right to refuse, but then you can continue to communicate therapeutically to assess the situation and negotiate a mutual goal.

There are also implications for communication with other health team members. You must learn to pose questions very clearly—and give answers that are equally clear. Be sure to ask other healthcare providers for their opinions on a problem. Don't make it seem that you want them to make decisions for you, but that you want their insights into the problem or how to solve it.

CONVERSATIONAL RITUALS

Many women aim to be liked by peers, and they use more conversational rituals than men do. Rituals focus on establishing symmetrical connections in relationships because of a need to be closely affiliated with peers. Many women attempt to maintain equality, make other people feel comfortable, look closely at the effects of conversations on a person's verbal and nonverbal behaviors, and maintain attention to details.

For example, many women say "I'm sorry" as a way of showing empathy and restoring balance to a conversation, not intending it to mean that they did something wrong. To some men, the woman who uses this phrase often may appear powerless. He may find himself wondering, "What is she sorry for?"

Another ritual for many women is use of the word "Thanks." The word "Thanks" is often tacked on to the end of a conversation, although there may be nothing to be thankful about. It is seen as a way of showing concern for others' feelings or work, and also as being kind and thanking them for their time. A man may wonder, "What is she thanking me for?"

A third ritual used by women is giving praise through compliments. Women offer more compliments than men, and they give far more compliments to other women than they do to men. It is a special form of feedback. Although people like to be praised, however, it gets annoying if it becomes habitual.

Men also use conversational rituals, many of which relate to status. Male rituals involve joking, sarcasm, teasing, and playful put-downs. To other men, this joking and teasing is part of the contest for status and a way of getting attention from others. Joking and teasing may also help avoid confronting an issue in an open manner. Women typically tell fewer jokes than men, and usually don't find teasing, sarcasm, and put-downs to be funny. Indeed, many women find certain types of humor destructive to relationships.

Nurses and Rituals

Examine your use of rituals. If you hear yourself saying, "I'm sorry," "Thank you," or offering compliments frequently and without a good reason for it, stop using these rituals. In addition, examine your use of joking. It can be useful in establishing rapport because everyone likes to laugh. However, sarcasm, teasing, and put-downs may not be taken as humorous, so be careful how you use humor in clinical situations. Encouraging emotional release using humor is the focus of Chapter 7.

Gender Differences in Nonverbal Behavior

Both men's and women's body language can be misinterpreted. Many women tend to have less confident body language and posture. Many women have been noted to take up less space, invade personal space less often, gesture more fluidly, and lower their eyes more in a negative encounter. This gives the impression of insecurity. They may also open their eyes wide to make a point, giving the impression of being naïve.[12] Women also smile and nod their heads more than men do. They tend to sit closer and look directly at each other as they speak.[2]

Many men, on the other hand, typically don't make direct facial contact with their eyes. They sit farther apart, at angles, and don't look at each other. To women, this gives the impression that men aren't paying attention or don't think the conversation is important. Men also touch women more often than women touch men.[14]

NURSES AND BODY LANGUAGE

Patients watch your body language closely, whether they know it or not. You must learn to project confidence and interest through your body language. Sit or stand 2 to 4 feet from the person, look at the person directly as you speak to him, and look into his eyes as you ask, "How are you doing today?" Listen carefully as he tells you. Watch his nonverbal behaviors. Smile and nod your head, as appropriate, in response to what the patient tells you. Touch is a special form of therapeutic communication involving body language and is the subject of Chapter 6.

Gender Responses to Discomfort

Of special concern to nurses are gender differences in responding to discomfort and physical health problems. Women are typically more expressive of discomforts and ask more questions than men. Many women tell you their discomforts. Many men may not volunteer information; during interviews, you may need to question them carefully to obtain the details of a problem. All patients, regardless of setting, should be carefully instructed to report discomforts and encouraged to take pain medications.

For example, suppose that you're assigned to a male patient who had a colon resection yesterday. He is refusing his pain medication because he says he doesn't need it. You go to change his dressing and find that he's rigid in the bed, his pulse and blood pressure are increased, and he winces and moans as you touch the tape on the dressing. You stop and say, "I can see this really hurts." He says, "I don't want to be a baby about pain." You explain that abdominal surgery is very painful and that the medication will ease the pain, making the dressing change much easier. In addition, you explain that he'll be able to move around better and be better able to prevent complications, such as pneumonia. He agrees to a pain medication.

To some men, illness may be viewed as taking away independence and status. As a result, they may ignore symptoms. They are

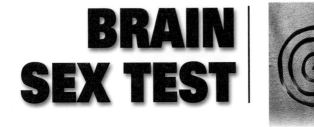

BRAIN SEX TEST

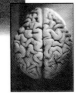

It is possible to test how male or female your own mind is.

The extent to which men and women exhibit masculine or feminine behavior is dependent on the organization of the brain into male or female patterns.

It is possible to be female and have some male mind attributes, and this simply depends on the presence or absence of the male hormone during certain stages of pregnancy.

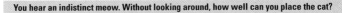

You hear an indistinct meow. Without looking around, how well can you place the cat?

(a) If you think about it you can point to it.
(b) You can point straight to it.
(c) You don't know if you could point to it.

How good are you at remembering a song you've just heard?

(a) You find it easy and you can sing part of it in tune.
(b) You can do it only if it's simple and rhythmical.
(c) You find it difficult.

A person you've met a few times telephones you. How easy is it for you to recognize the voice in the few seconds before the person tells you who he or she is?

(a) You'd find it quite easy.
(b) You'd recognize the voice at least half the time.
(c) You'd recognize the voice less than half the time.

You're with a group of married friends. Two of them are having a clandestine affair. Would you detect their relationship?

(a) Nearly always.
(b) Half the time.
(c) Seldom

You're at a large and purely social gathering. You're introduced to five strangers. If their names are mentioned the following day, how easy is it for you to picture their faces?

(a) You'll remember most of them.
(b) You'll remember a few of them.
(c) You'll seldom remember any of them.

In your early school days, how easy was spelling and the writing of essays?

(a) Both were quite easy.
(b) One was easy.
(c) Neither was easy.

Moir, A, and Jessel, D: Brain Sex: The Real Difference Between Men and Women. A Lyle Stuart Book published by Carole Publishing Group, Seacaucus: New Jersey, 1991.

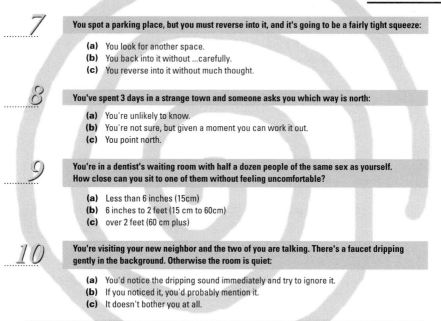

7

You spot a parking place, but you must reverse into it, and it's going to be a fairly tight squeeze:

(a) You look for another space.
(b) You back into it without ...carefully.
(c) You reverse into it without much thought.

8

You've spent 3 days in a strange town and someone asks you which way is north:

(a) You're unlikely to know.
(b) You're not sure, but given a moment you can work it out.
(c) You point north.

9

You're in a dentist's waiting room with half a dozen people of the same sex as yourself. How close can you sit to one of them without feeling uncomfortable?

(a) Less than 6 inches (15cm)
(b) 6 inches to 2 feet (15 cm to 60cm)
(c) over 2 feet (60 cm plus)

10

You're visiting your new neighbor and the two of you are talking. There's a faucet dripping gently in the background. Otherwise the room is quiet:

(a) You'd notice the dripping sound immediately and try to ignore it.
(b) If you noticed it, you'd probably mention it.
(c) It doesn't bother you at all.

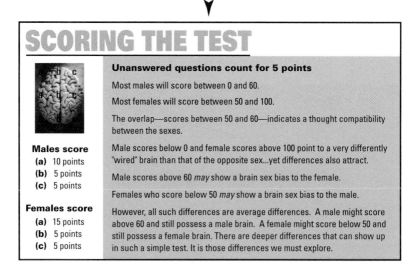

SCORING THE TEST

Unanswered questions count for 5 points

Most males will score between 0 and 60.

Most females will score between 50 and 100.

The overlap—scores between 50 and 60—indicates a thought compatibility between the sexes.

Males score
(a) 10 points
(b) 5 points
(c) 5 points

Females score
(a) 15 points
(b) 5 points
(c) 5 points

Male scores below 0 and female scores above 100 point to a very differently "wired" brain than that of the opposite sex...yet differences also attract.

Male scores above 60 *may* show a brain sex bias to the female.

Females who score below 50 *may* show a brain sex bias to the male.

However, all such differences are average differences. A male might score above 60 and still possess a male brain. A female might score below 50 and still possess a female brain. There are deeper differences that can show up in such a simple test. It is those differences we must explore.

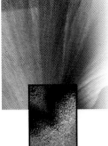

SEX TALK Quiz

		TRUE	FALSE
1	Women are more intuitive than men. They have a sixth sense, which is typically called "women's intuition."	[ ]	[ ]
2	At business meetings, co-workers are more likely to listen to men than they are to women.	[ ]	[ ]
3	Women are the "talkers." They talk much more than men in group conversations.	[ ]	[ ]
4	Men are the "fast talkers." They talk much faster than women.	[ ]	[ ]
5	Men are more outwardly open. They use more eye contact and exhibit more friendliness when first meeting someone.	[ ]	[ ]
6	Women are more complimentary. They give more praise than men.	[ ]	[ ]
7	Men interrupt more and will answer a question even when it is not addressed to them.	[ ]	[ ]
8	Women give more orders and are more demanding in the way they communicate.	[ ]	[ ]
9	In general, men and women laugh at the same things.	[ ]	[ ]
10	When making love, both men and women want to hear the same things from their partner.	[ ]	[ ]
11	Men ask for assistance less often than women do.	[ ]	[ ]
12	Men are harder on themselves and blame themselves more often than women.	[ ]	[ ]
13	Through their body language, women make themselves less confrontational than men.	[ ]	[ ]
14	Men tend to explain things in greater detail when discussing an incident.	[ ]	[ ]
15	Women tend to touch others more often than men.	[ ]	[ ]
16	Men appear to be more attentive than women when they are listening.	[ ]	[ ]
17	Women and men are equally emotional when they speak.	[ ]	[ ]
18	Men are more likely to discuss personal issues.	[ ]	[ ]

		TRUE	FALSE
19	Men bring up more topics of conversation.	[ ]	[ ]
20	Today, we tend to raise our male children the same way we do our female children.	[ ]	[ ]
21	Women tend to confront problems more directly and are likely to bring up the problem first.	[ ]	[ ]
22	Men are livelier speakers who use more body language and facial animation.	[ ]	[ ]
23	Men ask more questions than women.	[ ]	[ ]
24	In general, men and women enjoy talking about similar things.	[ ]	[ ]
25	When asking whether their partner has had an AIDS test or in discussing safe sex, a woman will likely bring up the topic before a man.	[ ]	[ ]

Glass, L: *He Says, She Says: Closing the Communication Gap Between the Sexes,* Berkley, New York, NY, 1992.

strong and can tough it out—no amount of pain or discomfort will keep them down. However, the risk of death is higher for males at all ages and from all leading causes.[15,16] Some men may need to become more in tune with what their bodies are telling them and seek help sooner.

Women, however, have a life expectancy that is 7 years longer than that of men. They restrict their activities for health problems 25 percent more days per year than men, and they spend 40 percent more days in bed per year than men. In middle and older age groups, women report more trouble performing activities, such as shopping, because of chronic health problems than men. Women older than age 45 also have up to 20 percent more physician visits, and obtain more prescriptions per year than men.[15,16] Women functioning in an affiliative manner may want the sympathy and support of healthcare providers and, consequently, willingly seek assistance.

SUMMARY

As a nurse, you need to become aware of communication differences based on gender and culture so that you can clearly deliver and decipher messages. Gender and family backgrounds are important to assess and consider in planning care for your patients. It makes a difference to understand that many women may be focused on affiliation, whereas many men may be focused on independence and status through their speech and body language during conversations. You must also become aware of your own cultural values, attitudes, and practices and how they affect your patient interactions.

Every nurse must become culturally sensitive and respect the beliefs, values, and practices of each patient's culture. You must learn to focus on developing rapport and trusting relationships as you assist the patient to attain an optimal level of well being or a peaceful death. You may need to modify your customary communication habits to avoid being misinterpreted and to deliver clear messages to patients and other healthcare providers. As you develop a better awareness of your personal cultural beliefs and communication patterns, you can modify and change your behavior to accommodate patients' health-related needs and better communicate with other healthcare providers.

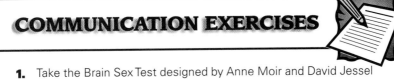

COMMUNICATION EXERCISES

1. Take the Brain Sex Test designed by Anne Moir and David Jessel shown on pages 55–56.[5] It will help you see how "male" or "female" your mind is regarding its organization into male or female patterns.

2. Take the Sex Talk Quiz designed by Lillian Glass shown on pages 57–58.[13] It shows some of what you know about current research on communications with the opposite sex. Correct answers to the quiz are 1. F; 2. T; 3. F; 4. F; 5. F; 6. T; 7. T; 8. F; 9. F; 10. F; 11. T; 12. F; 13. T; 14. F; 15. F; 16. F; 17. T; 18. F; 19. F; 20. F; 21. T; 22. F; 23. F; 24. F; 25. T.

3. The questions on pages 35–38 can help to guide a self-assessment of your cultural background. After you answer the questions for yourself, ask the questions of your parents and, if possible, your grandparents. After doing the assessment of your family's cultural background, compare and contrast your cultural background with that of classmates in small group discussions.

References

1. Hyde, JS: Half the Human Experience, ed 5. Houghton-Mifflin, Wilmington, Massachusetts, 1996.
2. Tannen, D: You Just Don't Understand: Women and Men in Conversation. Ballantine, New York, 1990.
3. Brannon, L: Gender: Psychological Perspectives. Allyn and Bacon, Boston, 1999.
4. Kozier, B, Erb, G, and Blais, K: Concepts and Issues in Nursing Practice, ed 2. Addison-Wesley, Redwood City, California, 1992.
5. Moir, A, and Jessel, D: Brain Sex: The Real Difference Between Men and Women. A Lyle Stuart Book published by Carole Publishing Group, Seacaucus: New Jersey, 1991.
6. Gorski, RA: Sexual Differentiation of the Endocrine Brain and Its Control Brain Endocrinology, ed 2. Raven Press, New York, 1991.
7. Lehne, RA: Pharmacology for Nursing Care, ed 3. WB Saunders, Philadelphia, 1998.
8. Gray, J: Men are from Mars, Women are from Venus. HarperCollins, New York, 1992.
9. Trossman, S. The human connection: Nurses and their patients. The American Nurse 30:1, DC 1998.
10. Lever, J. Sex differences in the complexity of children's play and games. American Sociological Review 43:471, 1978.
11. West, C and Zimmerman, DH: Small insults: A study of interruptions in cross-sex conversations between unacquainted persons. In Thorne, B, Kramarae, C, and Henley, N (eds). Language, Gender, and Society. Newbury House, Rowley, Massachusetts, 1983, p 103.
12. Burnside, I, and Haight, B: Reminiscence and life review: Therapeutic interventions for older people. Nurse Practitioner 19:55, 1994.
13. Glass, L: He Says, She Says: Closing the Communication Gap Between the Sexes. Berkley, New York, 1992.
14. Aries, E: Gender and Communication. In Shaver, P, and Hendrick, C (eds): Sex and Gender. Sage, Newbury Park, California, 1987, p 149–176.
15. Verbrugge, LM: Gender and health: An update on hypotheses and evidence. Journal of Health and Social Behavior 26:156, 1985.
16. Verbrugge, LM: The twain meet: Empirical explanations of sex differences in health and mortality. Journal of Health and Social Behavior 30:282, 1989.

Understanding the Effects of Self-Esteem and Body Image on Communication

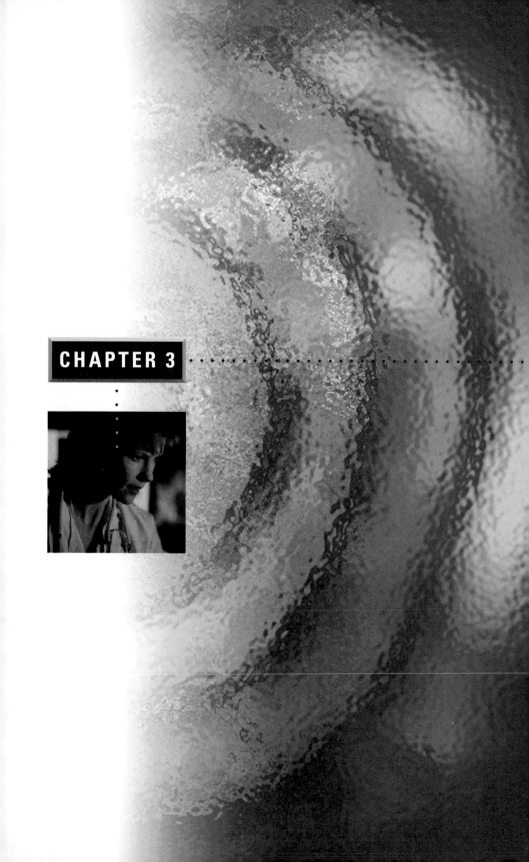

CHAPTER 3

Understanding the Effects of Self-Esteem and Body Image on Communication

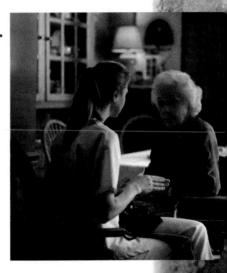

Chapter Objectives

AFTER READING THIS CHAPTER,
YOU WILL BE ABLE TO:

1. Define self-esteem and body image.
2. Identify the effects of self-esteem and body image on communication.
3. List factors that influence self-esteem and body image.
4. Examine the relationship between self-esteem and typical styles of communication.
5. Discuss how to build self-esteem in yourself and others.
6. Describe how to project a professional image.

THE PURPOSE OF THIS CHAPTER IS TO EXAMINE THE NATURE OF SELF-esteem and body image and how these concepts affect communication, therapeutic and otherwise. Self-esteem is the worth or value you place on yourself. Your level of self-esteem affects the words you speak and your nonverbal behaviors, including your facial expressions, tone of voice, gestures, and body positions. An important factor affecting self-esteem is the way you feel about your physical appearance, or body image.

To communicate effectively with patients and other healthcare providers, you'll want to create a positive impression by presenting a professional image. That image includes having a polished appearance, an authoritative voice, and a confident manner built on feelings of high self-esteem.

Self-Esteem

Virginia Satir's insights into self-esteem and communication will be a central focus of this chapter.[1] Satir suggests that the way a person communicates and interacts with others reflects the value that person places on himself. Your body language, tone of voice, and the words you use convey the positive or negative feelings and ideas you have about yourself. Examples of self-esteem and the value you place on yourself include feelings of being effective or ineffective, productive or worthless, capable or incapable, and likable or unlikable.

A person who likes himself can meet the challenges of life head-on, has realistic expectations of outcomes, and acts in an appropriate, effective, and responsible manner. He treats himself with dignity and respect. Those with high self-worth are better able to effectively communicate with others. That's because high self-esteem allows direct, clear, honest communication. The person can respond to others receptively, really listen to what others are saying, and treat others with respect. He can ask for advice and help from others but also can make his own decisions. A person with high self-esteem isn't afraid to fail. Indeed, he believes that he can learn from his mistakes.

When a crisis happens to someone with high self-esteem, the person will naturally feel disappointed and sad for a time. However, the person realizes that these feelings are temporary and need not be hidden. He still thinks of himself as having value and worth. He can level with others and talk openly about his feelings with people he trusts. A person with high self-esteem gives a whole-hearted effort and believes that he can reach the goal.

In contrast, low self-esteem exacts a high price. With low self-esteem, communication is indirect, vague, and dishonest. The person responds to others fearfully, he feels tension and stress, and he may end up placating or blaming others. The net effect of placating or blaming is that others don't like to be around a person perceived to be negative and not fun. As a result, the person with low self-esteem can be lonely and isolated.

When a person with low self-esteem experiences a crisis, he becomes fearful and unable to look objectively at the situation. He thinks, "This shows how worthless I really am. That's why these things always happen to me, and I have no control over them." Fear narrows a person's ability to perceive things clearly and keeps the person from carefully examining problems and possible solutions. This person fears failure and may become apathetic and indifferent. On the other hand, he may lash out at others during times of stress. Blaming and placating actually are attempts to cover up feelings of low self-esteem. The person who blames and placates can't discuss his feelings openly and honestly because it's too painful, he's afraid, and he believes that no one would understand even if he did talk to them.

A person with low self-esteem puts little effort into attaining goals. As a result, of course, he continues to fail, mainly from lack of effort. He says to himself, "I've failed before and I'll fail again." If the person doesn't keep trying, however, he can't grow. A vicious circle develops, with low self-esteem leading to poor communication, poor performance, a distorted view of self and others, and an unhappy personal life. Thus, self-esteem may decline even more.

Self-esteem is learned, and therefore, it constantly changes over time and with new experiences. Positive experiences increase self-esteem, and negative experiences decrease self-esteem. Feelings of worth can grow in any nurturing environment. The environment must be one in which each individual is treated with respect and individual differences are appreciated. Rules that you live by must be flexible. Communication is open and honest, and people trust each other and speak openly and honestly with each other, actively listening to each other. Everyone in the environment accepts responsibility for their mistakes, and mistakes are used for learning. Anyone can ask for help and get input into a problem but then make their own decisions. In addition, everyone in this environment has the right to change his mind. As you work with patients and establish relationships, the goal is to provide a nurturing environment to promote self-esteem in your patients.

Socialization: From ver did you come?

Were you raised in a nurturing environment? If so, you were probably raised by people who had high self-esteem. Your personal self-esteem was first influenced by your family experiences. It involved your interactions with significant others, such as parents, siblings, and grand-parents. From infancy, the words, looks, and touches from your family sent messages to build positive or negative self-esteem. These feelings went with you as you went to school. School experiences with teach-ers and classmates, your schoolwork, and extracurricular activities—such as sports—were next. When you became an adult, your job rela-tionships, including hirings, firings, promotions, and the ability to support your family and yourself affect your self-esteem. In addition, social groups throughout life, such as friends, neighbors, clubs, and hobbies affect your self-esteem.

Throughout life, a person with high self-esteem can handle many failures and retain the courage to make behavioral changes. But the person with low self-esteem, even with numerous successes, gives herself little credit for her accomplishments. She still has fear and self-doubts. She devalues herself and inflates her failures out of proportion to reality.

The poem by Satir on page 67 eloquently illustrates the concept of self-esteem.[2] Satir makes some excellent points in the poem, but above all, the poem shows the need for developing a "think positive" attitude. You must get to know yourself, and identify and accept your strengths and weaknesses. Everyone has both. You must set realistic goals and meet them by learning new skills and developing your abili-ties. You must take pride in your achievements, big and small; enjoy them; and give yourself lots of praise. You must take some time to be alone and enjoy your own company doing something you like to do, such as reading, exercising, or making something. You can learn to trust yourself by paying attention to your thoughts and feelings, and by acting on what you think is right and what makes you happy and ful-filled. Respect yourself. Be proud of who you are, and appreciate your own talents. Love yourself for the unique person you are. Learn to ac-cept your failures along with your successes. Does this mean that you'll become self-centered, egotistical, or snobbish? No. These nega-tive traits are false fronts for those with low self-esteem.

Communication Styles of People with Low Self-Esteem

The communication styles of people with low self-esteem were first described in chapter 1, and will be expanded upon now. These styles include the Placater, the Blamer, the Computer, and the Distracter. These styles of communication are attempts to cover up feelings of isolation, helplessness, incompetence, or feeling unloved as a reaction to the stress of a situation. The stress becomes an attack on self-

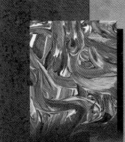

SELF ESTEEM

Virginia Satir

I am me.

In all the world, there is no one else like me.

There are persons who have some parts like me, but no one adds up exactly like me.

Therefore, everything that comes out of me is authentically mine because I alone chose it.

Therefore, everything about me
my body, including everything it does; my mind, including all its thoughts and ideas; my eyes, including the images of all they behold; my feelings, whatever they may be - anger, joy, frustration, love, disappointment, excitement; my mouth, and all the words that come out of it, polite, sweet or rough, correct or incorrect; my voice, loud or soft; and all my actions, whether they be to others or to myself.

I own my fantasies, my dreams, my hopes, my fears.

I own all my triumphs and successes, all my failures and mistakes.

Because I own all of me, I can become intimately acquainted with me.

By so doing I can love me and be friendly with me in all my parts.

I can then make it possible for all of me to work in my best interests.

I know there are aspects about myself that puzzle me, and other aspects that I do not know.

But as long as I am friendly and loving to myself, I can courageously and hopefully look for the solutions to the puzzles and for ways to find out more about me.

However I look and sound, whatever I say and do, and whatever I think and feel at a given moment in time is me.

This is authentic and represents where I am at that moment in time.

When I review later how I looked and sounded, what I said and did, and how I thought and felt, some parts may turn out to be unfitting.

I can discard that which is unfitting, and keep that which proved fitting and invent something new for that which I discarded.

I can see, hear, feel, think, say and do.

I have the tools to survive, to be close to others, to be productive and to make sense and order out of the world, of people and things outside of me.

I own me, and therefore I can engineer me.

I am me and I am okay.

esteem. When people use these patterns, they are really thinking, "I am unlovable and nobody cares about me. I have to act this way because it is how I am. I need to do this to survive."

The Placater believes that she must keep everyone happy so that she'll be liked or loved. She wants to do whatever another person wants just to make that person happy and keep that person from getting mad. The Placater experiences guilt, pity, and sometimes contempt for the person she is placating. The Placater tries to please to get on the person's good side, not because she really wants to do it. The Placater is rationalizing, "It is selfish not to do what is being asked."

The Blamer believes that, by yelling and giving orders, she is strong and in control of the situation. If she didn't fill that role, she thinks, nobody would do a thing. Underneath this exterior is a person who believes she is unloved and nobody cares about her. By getting someone to obey, she thinks she counts for something, which bolsters poor self-esteem. However, blaming makes the other person feel fearful, helpless, and resentful. Meanwhile, the Blamer is rationalizing, "I won't let anyone put me down. I won't be a coward."

The super-reasonable Computer needs to let everyone know that he's smart. The Computer wants you to believe that logic and ideas are all that count, and that emotions are a sign of weakness. Although this person looks calm and collected on the outside, inside he feels vulnerable and weak. The Computer makes the other person feel inferior, stupid, bored, and frustrated. The computer is rationalizing, "I'm not stupid. I'm too smart to make a mistake."

The Distracter tries to get attention through disruption. She doesn't focus on the topic of the conversation, and what she does and says doesn't make sense. She, too, believes that nobody cares about her. In conversation with a Distracter, the other person feels off balance, angry, and rejected. The Distracter is rationalizing, "It's not good to be so serious. We should live it up."

All of these communication styles drive others away rather than bringing them closer. These styles damage relationships. They're dishonest and hide our true feelings. The Placater hides her needs, the Blamer hides her need for the other person, the Computer hides his emotional needs, and the Distracter ignores her needs. These styles are used to cover up real feelings in a futile attempt to feel good about oneself.

The person using any of these styles is incongruent. Her feelings don't match her verbal and nonverbal behaviors. Thus the receiver gets a mixed message. People who use these styles may not be aware of what they're doing or why. They may be out of touch with themselves. Recognizing a problem in communication is the first step in making a change. We can all choose to do things differently and learn new ways to communicate. The goal is to become a congruent leveler, as described in the next section.

The Congruent Leveler

We all need to please others, criticize others, not get stepped on by others, and use our intellect to explain to others and change the subject when appropriate. A leveler can communicate effectively to accomplish all of these things. While leveling, you apologize for something you've done incorrectly or failed to do. When you criticize, you evaluate an act rather than blaming the person, and you make suggestions for better future performances. You can show your feelings as you give an explanation. You can also clearly say that you need to change the subject without confusing the other person as to what you are talking about.

The Leveler is also typically known throughout most of the nursing literature as an assertive person.[3-5] He delivers congruent messages. This means that his feelings and his verbal and nonverbal messages are matched. The Leveler asserts himself in a direct, honest, appropriate manner that doesn't interfere with another person's freedoms and rights.

Leveling is possible only when you recognize that everyone has personal rights and freedoms. General personal rights include the right to be treated with respect, to be listened to and taken seriously, and to change one's mind.[6] Personal freedoms include the freedom to say what you feel and think, the right to feel whatever you are feeling, and the right to ask for what you want. In your professional role, you have the right to a reasonable workload, the right to question or challenge, the right to make a mistake, and the right to do health teaching, as delineated in the Nurses Bill of Rights.[4] Recognition of your personal and professional rights is the first step toward learning to express yourself more effectively.

Nurses have had difficulties in expressing themselves in many situations, perhaps partially because of gender differences in communication. Chapter 2 mentioned that many women have been socialized to avoid conflict. In the past, nurses (who have been primarily female) have been trained to be submissive and to not rock the boat, that physicians (who have been primarily male) were more knowledgeable and powerful, and had to be obeyed. In the past, nurses were taught to stand when a physician entered the nurses' station. They even gave up seats where they had been working so the physician could sit down. Nurses who remain in such a submissive role may need to learn a more assertive, leveling communication style.

Perhaps because of the effects of these older role patterns, some nurses in more recent times have become defensive and aggressive. These nurses may need to learn to manage adversity with less aggressive responses. Therefore, a special emphasis is placed on communication skills in nursing programs.

If you're like most people, you probably will find it difficult to change your communication pattern because you fear negative consequences. You need to examine carefully these fears and develop new attitudes so you can become a Leveler. Leveling is an essential ingredient of therapeutic communication with patients and of effective communication with other health professionals—including physicians. You may fear making mistakes, being imperfect, or someone not liking what you do or thinking that you are no good. You may not like being criticized. You may feel that you're imposing on someone else. Also, you may fear retaliation.

Satir suggests that these attitudes need to be modified so that you can develop a positive outlook on life. This positive outlook will shine through in the way you communicate with others. She believes we should recognize that everyone makes mistakes because no one is perfect. Making mistakes is a part of every person's life. There will always be someone who doesn't like what you do; not everyone likes the same things. Also remember that everyone can use a little criticism, especially considering the fact that none of us are perfect. In addition, you impose on someone else each time you speak and interrupt with another person present. Finally, in response to a situation in which retaliation occurs, you can seek legal counsel or you can leave and find a better situation.

Styles of Communication in Nursing

In the vast majority of situations, the most effective style of communication involves a highly developed ability to level with others. The Leveler responds honestly and directly by telling someone what is wrong, why it's wrong, and what to do instead. Focus on the person's immediate actions that have upset you. First, tell the person what's wrong by explaining your true feelings. Say that you are angry, upset, sad, overwhelmed, or stressed out. Don't blame others by saying, "You make me so angry." Instead, replace "you" words with "I."

Next, tell the person why you feel the way you do by describing the situation. "I am angry about how long your break was. I've been having a very difficult time trying to manage my assignment and yours. We agreed that everyone would take only 10 minutes because we are short-staffed today, and you've been gone 30 minutes."

Last, tell the person what to do instead of the current behavior. This involves what you expect next time, as well as consequences if the behavior continues. "If you do not agree to abide by the schedule, I will refuse to take care of your patients for you while you are on break next time."

People who communicate using the other styles wouldn't be nearly so direct. For example, the Placater wouldn't say anything even though she was annoyed about what happened. She would avoid a confrontation to maintain harmony and avoid rocking the boat. This is the path of least resistance. She'd say something like, "Everything up here went fine while you were gone, no problem."

The Blamer would say, "What took you so long? What is the matter with you anyway? I was up here going crazy trying to care for my patients and yours. How selfish of you! Don't ever ask me to look after your patients while you take a break again!"

The Computer might say, "We must take many factors into consideration as we go on break. The care that the patients receive may be placed in jeopardy when the staff is short. Have you considered the risk to your health without a long break? I am sure there is a logical way to proceed; we need to talk more about these items."

The Distracter would say, "Hope you had a nice trip. Everything's okay up here. What's on the menu for lunch?"

Satir suggests that, in stressful interpersonal confrontational situations, 50 percent of people placate, 30 percent blame, 15 percent compute, and 0.5 percent distract to cope with the stress.[1] Only 4.5 percent of people are on the level. Learning to level takes practice. You've almost certainly been in situations that have made you angry and later devised what would have been the perfect thing to say to the other person. At the time, though, you said nothing. Or perhaps you blasted the other person and later wished that you had controlled yourself better. It takes practice to learn leveling, which is also known as assertiveness. Using the right words and behaviors to manage situations is a focus of Chapters 4 and 5.

The Leveler uses a communication pattern that demonstrates high self-esteem. He recognizes a problem and tries to confront the problem with a direct and honest approach. Leveling also yields even higher levels of self-esteem. Most people respect and admire others who have the courage to speak their minds, even when they do not agree with what the other person says.

Developing High Self-Esteem in Ourselves and Others

Building high self-esteem in yourself and those around you contributes to successful communication. With high self-esteem, you have the courage to speak your mind. You can help yourself and others feel better about their value. As a healthcare professional, you want to think positive. Your positive attitude will rub off onto others.

To develop these qualities, it's important to cultivate relationships with people who make you feel good, not those who put you down. Likewise, encourage others and help them communicate their feelings. Don't put yourself or others down. Be patient with faults and weaknesses. All of us have them. Also, use the following strategies to help your patients increase their self-esteem.

DEFINE CLEAR AND REALISTIC GOALS

The first step in building self-esteem is to define your goals clearly and make sure those goals are realistic. Keep in mind that most people tend to generalize too much and think in nonspecific ways. First, ask something like, "How would you like to feel differently about yourself?" The patient might respond with something like, "I want to feel happier." This answer is nonspecific, so ask a more specific question, such as "How will you know when you are happier?" Then the patient might answer, "I'd be happier if I could just lose 20 pounds." Now you have a specific goal that you can work toward. If the person is overweight and it would be realistic for her to lose 20 pounds, you can help her with a plan involving diet and exercise. Turn a nonspecific feeling into a specific goal to work toward. Reaching a goal, no matter how small, is a boost to self-esteem.

HELP PATIENTS THINK CLEARLY

People with low self-esteem tend to be negative and irrational. For example, the patient may say, "I can't do anything right."

Be careful not to contradict the patient with a statement like, "Of course you can" because it's argumentative. Instead, try to focus on specific behaviors by saying something like, "What exactly did you not follow through on?"

If the patient responds with, "I didn't follow the diet they gave me at the nutrition center," you now have something to work on. With this response, you can now discuss the diet and whatever difficulties the patient encountered when trying to adhere to the diet.

GIVE POSITIVE FEEDBACK

Giving honest praise to people for what they do, such as reaching a goal, bolsters their self-esteem. However, the praise must be honest, positive feedback for a job that was well done. Say something like, "I think you did a fine job" when the person really did do a fine job.

ENCOURAGE POSITIVE SELF-AFFIRMATIONS

To help encourage positive self-affirmations, have the patient make a list of things that he likes about himself. Examples of positive affirmations might include, "I am honest. I am a loving person. I am a good cook." You could have the patient write these things down on index cards and read them every day. In addition, tell him to do something that he does well every day.

STOP NEGATIVE THINKING

To help a patient willfully stop negative thinking about herself, tell her to say no to negative thoughts. To do so, she should force herself to think about the present, right now, rather than the past whenever a negative thought crops up. Then she should force herself to think of something she did well.

VISUALIZATION EXERCISES

Teach your patient to perform visualization exercises during relaxation. For example, teach him to take slow, deep breaths while listening to relaxing music and visualizing doing something differently. The something should pertain to a specific goal. For example, the patient could visualize himself being assertive in a situation, what he will say and do, and the good feeling he'll have as a result of honestly expressing himself.

Naturally, these techniques that work to improve your patients' self-esteem can also work to improve your own. Take time to try them, and make note of the result.

Body Image

Body image is an important factor affecting self-esteem. Body image refers to feelings and attitudes about the physical body. These feelings and attitudes are based on perceptions you have formed about your physical characteristics. In addition, people around you affect how you think about your body. If you receive compliments about how you look, it reinforces the good feelings you have about you body. If

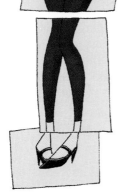

you believe you look good, you are probably also feeling good about yourself in general. Feeling good about yourself leads to confidence when you communicate with others. Research substantiates the fact that many of us do not feel good about some of the parts of our bodies that make up our physical appearance, as comically depicted by the cartoon on this page.[7]

Research indicates that 55 percent of the meaning we get from someone delivering a message is based on visual cues.[8] Bernscheid's research indicates that subjects viewing photographs judged attractive people to have more poise and sensitivity than people judged to be less attractive.[9] The subjects also rated people who looked attractive in pictures to be more sociable, outgoing, interesting, and stronger that those who looked less attractive to them. So, without a word being spoken, patients and other healthcare providers make many judgments about you, just based on your outward physical appearance.

Many of us are uncomfortable with some of the parts of our bodies that make up our physical appearance.

Have you ever noticed how successful people look successful? They know how to groom themselves and select clothes that look attractive on them. Research indicates that a professional image enhances your ability to communicate with other people.[10] Nurses have become concerned with creating positive impressions and projecting a professional image.[11] The idea of the professional image has been recognized as very important to the business executive. Both men and women in business have focused on how to dress and act for success in recent years.[12,13] Professional image consulting has become a large industry. Because many nurses no longer wear uniforms and serve in many different settings, there is similarity between professional business and professional nursing attire. Like business executives, nurses have come to recognize the effects of a professional image on communication.[11]

First, you need a realistic picture of your body and the bodies of other people. Only a very rare few have the bodies of models pictured in fashion magazines. Because so few of us are perfectly proportioned and the perfect weight, your goal is to create an attractive and professional image with the body you have. You can learn to select clothes that are flattering to your body build. For example, if you are smaller on the top half of your body than the bottom half, you can wear shoulder pads to make your hips look slimmer and give a more balanced appearance. If you have long legs, cuffed pants will appear to shorten them. If you have short legs, wearing pants without cuffs will give the illusion of longer legs. To appear taller and slimmer, you can buy clothing with vertical lines. If you're thin, you can wear clothing with horizontal lines to appear wider. Information on dressing for the size and shape of the body has been a popular topic of many books and professional journals.[12-16]

Color Analysis

You can also enhance your professional image by wearing colors that flatter the natural coloring of your skin, hair, and eyes.[15,16] This is true of both men and women. Women may choose to also include makeup in this color analysis.

The analysis is based on your skin's undertone, which is either warm (yellow) or cool (blue). These cool and warm tones are further divided into categories that are related to the seasons of the year. In other words, your coloring may make you a winter, a spring, a summer, or an autumn; winters and summers have cool undertones, and autumns and springs have warm undertones.

If you're a winter, you look best in clear primary colors, such as navy, black, white, red, shocking pink, and gray. Most people are categorized as winter. If you're a summer, you look best in soft pastels, such as light blue, rose brown, navy, rose pink, lavender, and plum.

Autumns look best in warm, rich, fall colors that have golden undertones, such as dark brown, camel, beige, orange gold, and moss green. Springs look best in golden brown, camel, peachy pink, peach, bright blues, and golden yellow. Many more colors are included in each category; however, those listed here give you the general idea that certain categories of colors are most flattering on people of certain skin tones.

The procedure to determine your season is to sit before a well-lighted mirror without any makeup on your skin and hold up different colors to your face. Determine which colors light up your skin, eyes, and hair, and which make you look washed out or give a yellow cast to your skin. For example, if a winter (typically a dark-haired person with very light skin) wears beige, it will make her look pale and give a yellow cast to her skin.

You may be interested in having an analysis done by a professional color consultant. This person can advise you on the many different colors in clothing and make-up that will most flatter you. You can also find more about color analysis and clothing selection in the references included at the end of the chapter.

Clothing Colors and Styles: What's Your Message?

The style and colors you wear send signals. They may be appropriate or inappropriate, helpful or not helpful, in establishing a professional image. As a general rule, the situation should dictate the color and style of the clothing you choose to wear.[10,13] The classic colors of professional business attire are black, navy blue, gray, and beige. Wear these colors to meetings. Strength and sincerity are associated with navy blue. Gray is a color of strength but also is a neutral color and sends a message of a more conservative and objective manner. Blue and gray are also good interview colors. Black suggests power and is dressier than navy or gray. Beige connotes authority and is a neutral and dispassionate color suggesting self-containment. Although brown is a dark color, it is associated with earth and lacks the power of black, navy, gray, or beige.

When you wear a bright color, such as red, you give the appearance of having energy and animation. It is an excellent color for making a speech or giving a presentation. Other intense colors, such as royal blue and purple, are associated with royalty. Emerald green expresses new life or regeneration, and gold is connected with wealth. Pastels are associated with innocence.

Some nurses continue to wear white uniforms and lab coats. White suggests clarity and crispness. Keep in mind, however, that white can have a cool (blue) cast or a warm (yellow) cast and includes anything from stark white to cream. Wear the color of white that goes best with your skin undertones.

The Nursing Dress Code

All nursing programs have a dress code for students, and working nurses typically have had to follow some form of dress code. More recently, nurses have come to focus on how they may effectively create professional images to communicate more clearly with patients and other healthcare providers.[11] The intent here is to expand on why the dress code is so important to follow.

A crisp and efficient appearance gives you an air of authority and orderliness. It suggests that you are in control of the situation. It means that you attend to details and builds confidence in patients and their families. Fresh, clean, ironed clothes are essential. The style of the clothing is also an important consideration. You may have a choice of uniform style and should adopt the style most flattering to your body. At least you may have a choice once you graduate. Some programs require the same uniform for all students. In any case, make sure the uniform is loose. If you're female, consider wearing pants, if you have a choice, because you'll be doing a lot of bending over and lifting. Always have your shoes clean and polished.

On some hospital units, you may wear a scrub uniform. If the colors of the standard issue scrub uniform are wrong for you, you can compensate by wearing flattering makeup. You may have a choice in the color of the cover-up jacket or sweater that can be worn over the uniform or scrub suit.

Even if you must wear a white lab coat, the clothes under the lab coat should be of a style and color that flatters you. Consider wearing simple, classic, comfortable styles in solid colors with clean lines under your lab coat. Avoid ruffles and bows; details on clothes can be distracting. The most professional-looking trousers or skirts should be in dark colors like black, navy, or brown. A shirt, blouse, or sweater in your best colors with a conservative neckline can be worn under the lab coat. Neckties or scarves should be conservative and in colors that are flattering to you. Wear a closed-toe, comfortable leather shoe that is conservative.

Keep jewelry to a minimum. Remember, however, that carefully selected jewelry can be attractive and give you a positive image. Gold or silver earrings that are close to the ear, such as balls, knots, or small hoops, are appropriate. Pins can also be worn on your uniform; these include your school pin, the sigma theta tau pin, or health awareness pins, such as breast cancer or acquired immunodeficiency syndrome (AIDS) pins. Pins can also serve as a point of light conversation with a patient as you establish rapport. If you wear a lab coat and street clothes, you might wear a pendant necklace or other conservative necklace to brighten your appearance.

Your hairstyle, along with makeup for women, form important components of the professional image. Heavy makeup and a dramatic hairstyle take away from the look of competence. Choose cosmetics that give a natural, fresh look and are in your colors. Keep your hair neat, glossy clean, and off your face. Clean, controlled hair means that you care about yourself and projects capability. If you have long hair, keep it in place with barrettes or combs in gold, silver, bronze, or white for a white uniform or a color to match your clothing under the lab coat. Frizzy hair styles, teased hair, and hair falling in your eyes is not appropriate, and not just for your image. Hair that's out of control

HOW DO YOU

SEE YOURSELF?

Purpose. This scale is designed to assist you in understanding your self-image. Positive attitudes toward oneself are important components of maturation and emotional well-being.

Directions. Read each statement carefully. Circle the letter in the columns on the right that corresponds to your response to each statement.

RATING

Strongly Agree
Agree
Disagree
Strongly Disagree

SELF-IMAGE ASPECT

1.	I feel that I'm a person of worth, at least on an equal plane with others.	A	B	C	D
2.	I feel that I have a number of good qualities.	A	B	C	D
3.	All in all, I am inclined to feel that I am a failure.	A	B	C	D
4.	I am able to do things as well as most other people.	A	B	C	D
5.	I feel I do not have as much to be proud of as others.	A	B	C	D
6.	I take a positive attitude toward myself.	A	B	C	D
7.	On the whole, I am satisfied with myself.	A	B	C	D
8.	I wish I could have more respect for myself.	A	B	C	D
9.	I certainly feel useless at times.	A	B	C	D
10.	At times I think I am no good at all.	A	B	C	D

SCORING

Use the following table to determine the number of points to assign to each of your answers. To determine your total score, add up all the numbers that match the letter (A,B,C, or D) you circled for each statement.

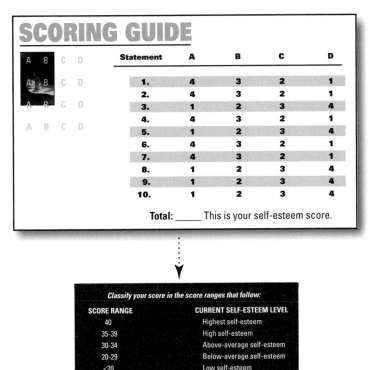

SCORING GUIDE

Statement	A	B	C	D
1.	4	3	2	1
2.	4	3	2	1
3.	1	2	3	4
4.	4	3	2	1
5.	1	2	3	4
6.	4	3	2	1
7.	4	3	2	1
8.	1	2	3	4
9.	1	2	3	4
10.	1	2	3	4

Total: _____ This is your self-esteem score.

Classify your score in the score ranges that follow:

SCORE RANGE	CURRENT SELF-ESTEEM LEVEL
40	Highest self-esteem
35-39	High self-esteem
30-34	Above-average self-esteem
20-29	Below-average self-esteem
<20	Low self-esteem

Interpretation. The higher you score, the more positive your self-esteem. High self-esteem means that individuals respect themselves, consider themselves worthy, but do not necessarily consider themselves better than others. They do not feel themselves to be the ultimate in perfection; on the contrary, they recognize their limitations and expect to grow and improve.

Self-esteem is the most important variable in regard to human development and maturation. It is the master key that can open the door to the actualization of an individual's human potential.

Making Changes: Boosting Self-Esteem

- Use affirmations, positive statements that help reinforce the most positive aspects of your personality and experience. Every day, you can boost your sense of esteem by saying positive things about you to yourself, such as "I am a loving, caring person," or "I am honest and open in expressing my feelings." You may want to write some affirmations of your own on index cards and flip through them occasionally.

- List the things you would like to have or experience. Construct the statements as if you were already enjoying the situations you list, beginning each sentence with "I am." For example, "I am feeling great about doing well in my classes," or "I am enjoying the opportunity to meet new people. "Visualize each situation, and get in the habit of repeating this process several times a day.

- When your internal critic—the negative inner voice we all have—starts putting you down, tune it out. Force yourself to think of a situation that you handled well or something about yourself that you're especially proud of.

A quiz to help you determine your self-esteem. (Adapted from Rosenberg, M: Society and the Adolescent Self-Image. Wesleyan University Press, Middletown, Connecticut, 1989.)

can be a source of infection for patients. If you have long hair that is not appropriately controlled and falls onto a patient as you lean over to do a procedure, you will probably receive a lecture on professional image and infection control from your clinical faculty. Loose hair should be no longer than the chin, and worn in a soft and sleek style.

In summary, colors, clothing styles, makeup, and hairstyles are important components of the professional image. These visual cues are important aspects of communication.

Posture

Posture is another important component of the professional image involving visual aspects of communication. Use good posture when sitting or standing. Keep your shoulders back and your spine straight. Remember that body language sends a strong message. An open, relaxed posture is appropriate. Sitting slouched in a chair, with your arms crossed or your body facing away from the other person, could send a message of boredom, lack of interest, even hostility. Also, avoid using mannerisms that distract from sending and receiving accurate messages. For example, twisting an earring, twisting your hair, biting your fingernails, and chewing your lip are all signs of nervousness that must be avoided.

Say It as Though You Mean It!

In addition to the way you look, the way you sound in the quality of your voice can also help you communicate more effectively.[12] Although looks account for 55 percent of a first impression, tone of voice accounts for 38 percent of that impression.[8] The aim is to project a "listen to me" voice that conveys conviction, energy, and confidence. The way your voice sounds is best revealed in a phone conversation. The way you sound on the phone creates a mental picture for the listener and suggests who you are. Your voice needs to convey interest, enthusiasm, and credibility.

Whether you are using the phone or talking face to face, if you speak softly, patients may think you don't believe what you are saying. That reduces your effectiveness. If you speak softly and with a breathy or shaky voice, people may get the impression that you lack power and authority, and that you're timid and weak. If you speak in a meek, childish voice, you won't sound like someone to be taken seriously. Therefore, if you have a soft voice, you can project confidence by smiling and learning to project your voice more powerfully than you nor-

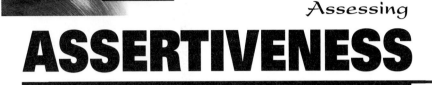

Assessing

ASSERTIVENESS

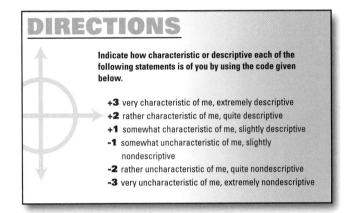

DIRECTIONS

Indicate how characteristic or descriptive each of the following statements is of you by using the code given below.

+3 very characteristic of me, extremely descriptive
+2 rather characteristic of me, quite descriptive
+1 somewhat characteristic of me, slightly descriptive
-1 somewhat uncharacteristic of me, slightly nondescriptive
-2 rather uncharacteristic of me, quite nondescriptive
-3 very uncharacteristic of me, extremely nondescriptive

_____ **1** Most people seem to be more aggressive and assertive than I am.*

_____ **2** I have hesitated to make or accept dates because of "shyness."*

_____ **3** When the food served at a restaurant is not done to my satisfaction, I complain about it to the waiter or waitress.

_____ **4** I am careful to avoid hurting other people's feelings, even when I feel that I have been injured.*

_____ **5** If a salesman has gone to considerable trouble to show me merchandise that is not quite suitable, I have a difficult time in saying "No."*

_____ **6** When I am asked to do something, I insist on knowing why.

_____ **7** There are times when I look for a good, vigorous argument.

_____ **8** I strive to get ahead as well as most people in my position.

_____ **9** To be honest, people often take advantage of me.*

_____ **10** I enjoy starting conversations with new acquaintances and strangers.

_____ **11** I often don't know what to say to attractive persons of the opposite sex.*

_____ **12** I hesitate to make phone calls to business establishments and institutions.*

_____ **13** I would rather apply for a job or for admission to a college by writing letters than by going through with personal interviews.*

_____ **14** I find it embarrassing to return merchandise.*

_____ **15** If a close and respected relative were annoying me, I would smother my feelings rather than express my annoyance.*

____ *16*   I have avoided asking questions for fear of sounding stupid.*

____ *17*   During an argument I am sometimes afraid that I will get so upset that I will shake all over.*

____ *18*   If a famed and respected lecturer makes a statement that I think is incorrect, I will have the audience hear my point of view as well.

____ *19*   I avoid arguing over prices with clerks and salesmen.*

____ *20*   When I have done something important or worthwhile, I manage to let others know about it.

____ *21*   I am open and frank about my feelings.

____ *22*   If someone has been spreading false and bad stories about me, I see him (her) as soon as possible to "have a talk" about it.

____ *23*   I often have a hard time saying "No."*

____ *24*   I tend to bottle up my emotions rather than make a scene.*

____ *25*   I complain about poor service in a restaurant and elsewhere.

____ *26*   When I am given a compliment, I sometimes just don't know what to say.*

____ *27*   If a couple near me in a theater or at a lecture were conversing rather loudly, I would ask them to be quiet or to take their conversation elsewhere.

____ *28*   Anyone attempting to push ahead of me in a line is in for a good battle.

____ *29*   I am quick to express an opinion.

____ *30*   There are times when I just can't say anything.*

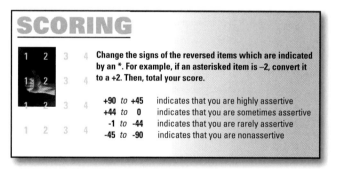

SCORING

Change the signs of the reversed items which are indicated by an *. For example, if an asterisked item is –2, convert it to a +2. Then, total your score.

+90 *to* **+45**	indicates that you are highly assertive
+44 *to* **0**	indicates that you are sometimes assertive
-1 *to* **-44**	indicates that you are rarely assertive
-45 *to* **-90**	indicates that you are nonassertive

A quiz to help you assess your level of assertiveness. (Adapted from Rathus, S: A 30-item schedule for assessing assertive behavior. Behavior Therapy 4:398–406, 1973. Reprinted with permission.)

mally would. There's a big difference in impression between hearing "We need to discuss this problem" in a strong, vibrant tone and hearing it in a meek, childish tone.

To check to determine whether or not you are projecting your voice, find the natural pitch of your voice by humming. Hum the notes in a scale. As you hum, whenever you hear vibrating or buzzing is the vocal range where your voice is strongest. Your speaking voice should be at the same pitch because the vibrating helps project the voice and adds authority.

Also, be sure not to raise the pitch of your voice at the end of a declarative sentence. If you do, you'll sound as though you're asking a question and are unsure of yourself. Instead, you want to sound authoritative, so practice lowering your voice at the end of a declarative sentence. Pauses at appropriate intervals act as vocal punctuation marks. Leave a brief moment of silence after an important thought to help the patient absorb your message easily. In addition, slow your speech and pronounce the words clearly.

The words we speak account for 7 percent of the message that is to be communicated.[8] Always choose your words carefully as you communicate. If you use disclaiming phrases, such as "I'm not sure," "This is only my opinion," and "This probably sounds dumb, but. . . ," you'll sound as though you lack confidence. In addition, avoid using slang. If you find some words difficult to pronounce, replace them with words that are easier to say but mean the same thing.

SUMMARY

The purpose of this chapter is to analyze the effects of self-esteem and body image on communication. Self-esteem is the general feeling of value and worth a person holds about himself. Body image is the personal view of the physical self, and is a key factor affecting self-esteem.

Self-esteem directly affects our basic style of communication. Lack of self-esteem leads to a lack of confidence in dealing with people, solving problems, and performing duties. It also gives a distorted view of the self and others. Poor self-esteem results in damaging communication patterns, such as blaming, placating, computing, and distracting. It takes a lot of self-esteem to use a therapeutic communication style of leveling consistently. Self-esteem can be improved by setting realistic goals, encouraging positive self-evaluations, using praise and self-affirmations, stopping negative thoughts, and performing visualization exercises. The goal is to make a habit of feeling good about yourself—and to help your patients do the same.

You must learn to create a positive professional image. The color and style of your clothes, hair, makeup, and jewelry can create this image. The projection of your voice and the words you speak are also important aspects of the total professional demeanor. Always remember the nonverbal way that you look and act conveys 55 percent of an initial impression, with the tone of voice accounting for 35 percent and the words you speak accounting for 7 percent of a message. Knowing you convey a professional image gives you confidence and enhances positive responses from patients and staff, which directly contributes to improved self-esteem.

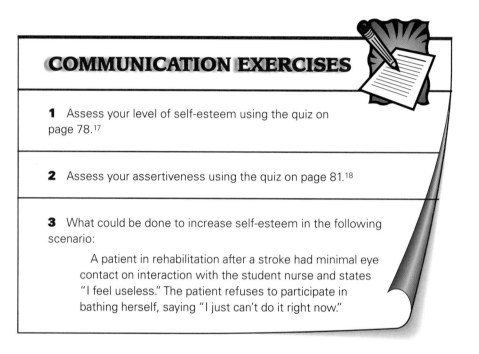

COMMUNICATION EXERCISES

1 Assess your level of self-esteem using the quiz on page 78.[17]

2 Assess your assertiveness using the quiz on page 81.[18]

3 What could be done to increase self-esteem in the following scenario:

> A patient in rehabilitation after a stroke had minimal eye contact on interaction with the student nurse and states "I feel useless." The patient refuses to participate in bathing herself, saying "I just can't do it right now."

References

1. Satir, V: The New Peoplemaking. Science and Behavior Books, Mountainview, California, 1988.
2. Satir, V: Self Esteem. Celestial Arts, Berkeley, California, 1970.
3. Angel, G, and Petronko, DK: Developing the new assertive nurse. Springer, New York, 1983.
4. Herman, SJ: Becoming Assertive: A Guide for Nurses. D. Van Nostrand, New York, 1978.
5. Clark, CC: Assertive Skills for Nurses. Contemporary Publishing, Wakefield, Massachusetts, 1978.
6. Bloom, LZ, Coburn, K, and Pearlman, J: The New Assertive Woman. Dell, New York, 1977.
7. Brannon, L: Gender: Psychological Perspectives. Allyn and Bacon, Boston, 1999.

8. Mehrabian, A: Nonverbal Communication. Aldine-Atherton, Inc, Chicago, Illinois, 1972.
9. Berscheid, E, and Walster, E: Physical attractiveness. In Berkowitz, L (ed). Advances in Experimental Social Psychology. Academic Press, New York, 1974.
10. Wallach, J: Looks that Work. Viking Penguin, New York, 1986.
11. Anderson, K: Creating a positive first impression. Nursing 98 *28*:60, 1998.
12. Sobkowski, A: How to project power. Executive Female 12(6):26, 1989.
13. Molloy, JT: The Woman's Dress for Success Book. Reardon and Walsh, Milwaukee, Wisconsin, 1977.
14. Abravanel, E, and King, E: Dr. Abravanel's Body Type Diet and Lifetime Nutrition Plan. Bantam Books, New York, 1983.
15. Jackson, C: Color Me Beautiful. Ballantine, New York, 1984.
16. Jackson, C: Color for Men. Ballantine, New York, 1984.
17. Rosenberg, M: Society and the Adolescent Self-Image. Wesleyan University Press, Middletown, Connecticut, 1989.
18. Rathus, S. A 30-item schedule for assessing assertive behavior. Behavior Therapy *4*:398, 1973.

Emotional Reactions to the Stress of Illness

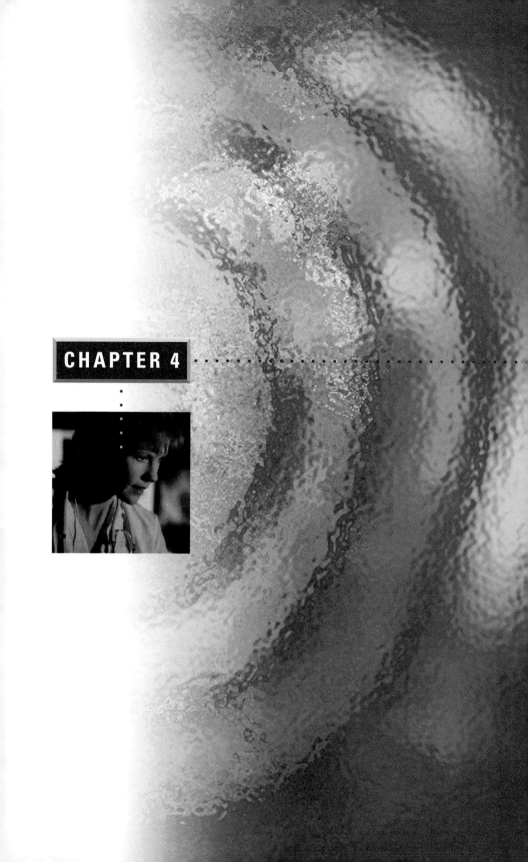

CHAPTER 4

Emotional Reactions to the Stress of Illness

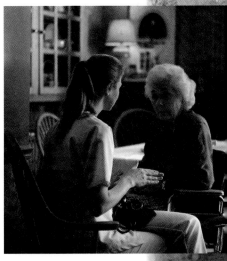

Chapter Objectives

AFTER READING THIS CHAPTER,
YOU WILL BE ABLE TO:

1. Describe the effect of illness on self-esteem.

2. List the typical stages of illness and relate them to emotional reactions.

3. Discuss the loss and grief responses during illnesses and life-changing conditions.

4. Examine the sick role and emotional reactions to dependency.

5. Identify the nontherapeutic effects of withholding emotions and the therapeutic effects of ventilating emotions.

6. Identify the therapeutic effects of emotional expression.

7. Differentiate between empathy and sympathy.

8. Describe typical blocks that downplay the emotional response during nurse-patient communication.

9. Describe typical facilitation techniques to encourage expression of emotions during nurse-patient communication.

10. Describe the nursing burnout syndrome and how to prevent it.

THE PURPOSE OF THIS CHAPTER IS TO FOCUS ON HOW EMOTIONAL REACtions to illness affect a person's ability to communicate. In addition, the chapter focuses on how to identify a patient's emotional response and how to use basic therapeutic communication techniques to help the person express emotions. The chapter also helps you develop an awareness of your own emotional responses in clinical situations and how they effect patients. Also, it helps you learn how to manage your personal emotional responses.

Illness: A Threat to Self-Esteem for Patient, Family, and Nurse

Patients and families have emotional reactions to illness because illness is a threat to self-esteem.[1] As defined in Chapter 3, self-esteem is the worth or value people place on themselves. Alterations in self-esteem occur during illness because of numerous threats inherent to illness, such as threats to livelihood, role performance, and even life itself.

The type of illness and the person's perception of its implications are two important factors that relate to the impact on self-esteem. Self-esteem declines because the person can't perform all the life activities he could formerly. Self-esteem also can be affected by alterations in body image, depending on the nature of the illness. For example, consider the 36-year-old woman who works as an elementary school teacher, has a husband and two young children, and has undergone a mastectomy. Her self-esteem will be affected—profoundly—by the change in her body image brought on by the mastectomy. Her self-esteem will also be affected by her reduced ability to perform her roles of teacher, wife, and mother.

As a nurse, your self-esteem may be affected as well by the emotional scenario described earlier. That's because you may have doubts about your ability to manage your own emotions and the emotional reactions of the patient and her family. Emotions are contagious; those felt by the patient and her family will be transmitted to you. For example, you may feel sad along with a patient and family who must face cancer and its treatment. You may expect yourself to be able to deal with emotions in yourself as well as in the patient and her family. However, if you feel inadequate to handle emotional responses to illness that you believe you should be able to manage effectively, your self-esteem may suffer and your level of anxiety will rise. In general, you'll feel anxious whenever you believe you should be able to perform a nursing intervention, but you don't in fact have the necessary knowledge and skill to do it.

The way to build self-esteem in yourself is to develop knowledge and competence in dealing with emotional tensions in patients, their families, and yourself. It requires high self-esteem for a nurse to remain calm and compassionate in the midst of human struggles that arise daily in healthcare situations.

Impact of Illness: Physical and Psychosocial Stages

The types and the ramifications of illness that affect a patient's self-esteem involve two components: physical and psychosocial.[2] Although these phases occur simultaneously, they're described separately here to facilitate your understanding of patient and family reactions to illness.

PHYSICAL STAGES

The physical stages of illness are its onset, course, and prognosis. An illness may have gradual *onset,* with symptoms getting progressively worse, as in diabetes, or it may have a sudden onset, as in a head injury that results from a car accident. *Course* refers to the length of time the person has to alter her lifestyle to manage the problem. A person with a broken leg usually must alter her lifestyle about two months with a cast and therapy. The person with chronic diabetes must make permanent changes in lifestyle.

Prognosis refers to the expected outcome, such as complete recovery, chronic illness, or death. For example, a person with a broken leg is expected to get completely better. A person with diabetes is expected to get better but must learn to manage blood sugar levels to attain an optimal level of functioning. A person with a serious head injury is expected to die within 24 hours. The physical states are clear and easily recognized.

PSYCHOSOCIAL STAGES

Much more complicated than the physical stages are the psychosocial, emotion-laden stages of illness. The emotional response to illness is an attempt to control damage done to self-esteem.

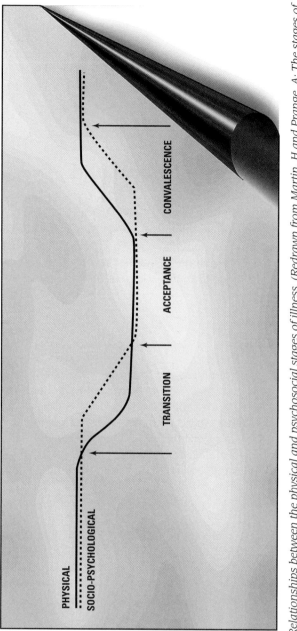

Relationships between the physical and psychosocial stages of illness. (Redrawn from Martin, H and Prange, A: The stages of illness: Psychosocial approach. Nurs Outlook 10(3):168–171, March, 1962. Reprinted with permission.)

PHYSICAL

SOCIO-PSYCHOLOGICAL

TRANSITION

ACCEPTANCE

CONVALESCENCE

The damage to self-esteem can be related to loss. The patient and family suffer losses when they may never be the same again as a result of the illness. The patient may lose a body part or a physiological function, such as the ability to have children after a hysterectomy. Illness may cause the patient to lose external possessions as well, such as his job. The patient and family may lose their home, for example, if illness requires that the patient be placed in a nursing home or extended-care facility. In addition, permanent neurological changes or death can take the patient, as they knew him, away from his family. For many of the changes brought about by illness, patients and families gradually adjust to the losses and damage to self-esteem.

Psychologically and socially, the patient and his family assimilate the physical changes by going through three phases: a transition to illness, acceptance of the illness, and convalescence as the patient recovers.[2] The relationships between the physical and psychosocial stages are shown in the figure on page 92.[2] This model shows that the sociopsychological transition to illness lags behind the physical state, often because the patient denies symptoms. During acceptance, the physical and sociopsychological states are in close correlation. In convalescence, the sociopsychological state may again lag behind the physical state, commonly because the patient feels insecure about his ability to perform all the activities that he used to do before the illness. In the event of significant loss, the patient and family will mourn the loss, and they may go through the stages of denial, anger, bargaining, depression, and acceptance.[3] If the patient dies, the family will experience grief and may go through these stages.

TRANSITION TO ILLNESS

The transition to illness is the time between the appearance of an illness (the onset) and the patient's admission to himself that he is indeed ill. The self-image of a healthy and vital person is being disrupted by symptoms. Denial and rationalization characterize this period; both are defenses against the threatened self-esteem. Both are done to avoid the emotions associated with becoming ill. The patient may say things to himself like, "This pain in my chest is just indigestion. I'll continue to shovel snow." Or he may say, "This can't be my heart because I've never had anything serious wrong with me." However, if the pain grows worse, radiating down his arms and into his jaw as he continues to shovel snow, and if he grows so short of breath that he fears he'll pass out, eventually he'll decide that it's time to go to the emergency room. He has made the transition to illness.

ACCEPTANCE

At the point when the person has decided something is definitely wrong and he needs to do something about it, he has entered the stage of acceptance. The patient may experience a wide range of feelings at this point depending on the extent of his illness and the effects he thinks it will have on his life. Let's continue with the above-mentioned patient who had a heart attack.

As this person begins to receive healthcare, he'll be afraid as healthcare professionals attach him to equipment and perform tests. He'll also be afraid of what might be ahead, such as surgery, pain, disfigurement, and even death. Fear disrupts the ability to think clearly and problem solve when reviewing options and deciding on a suitable course of treatment.

CONVALESCENCE

Convalescence begins once the patient is stabilized and starts to recover. Physically, he's getting better. Sadness and anger are prevalent in this stage. The patient may become frustrated and upset, especially if his illness is extended or severe. The limitations on functioning are the primary problem.

The damaged self-esteem is reflected in the statement, "I am not worth anything now that I can no longer. . . ." The independent and self-sufficient bank president who had a stroke may react angrily when being told what to do by healthcare providers. The construction foreman may feel sad about not being able to work any more after his heart attack because "I worked all my life." The mother of two young children is sad because she misses her children very much and is anxious about the care they're receiving while she recovers from her car accident. Each of these situations reflects the insecurity commonly felt by patients as they recover from serious illness.

GRIEF

Grief associated with death and significant loss initially produces shock, disbelief, and denial. As the loss begins to sink in, many people feel anger because they have no control over the situation. As a result, they may direct that anger at you or other healthcare personnel. Next, they may express guilt and fear that they're being punished. Depression and sadness occur when the patient and family recognize that their lives will never be the same again. Last, the patient and family come to terms with the loss and begin making plans.[3]

The Patient's Personal and Unique Response

Not everyone goes through each physical and psychosocial stage. Also, while in a stage, not everyone progresses at the same rate. In addition, not everyone responds in the same way during a stage. People's responses depend on their previous experience with illness and the healthcare system, as well as on their gender and cultural differences as described in Chapters 1 and 2. In general, the more severe the illness, the more extensive the emotional, behavioral, and physical response. However, two patients who have the same diagnosis may respond quite differently, sometimes unexpectedly, as depicted in the cartoon below.

You must become aware, however, that even a minor illness can cause emotional and physical reactions. Think of how true this is in

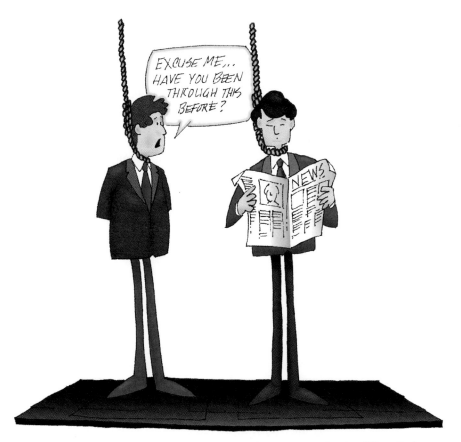

Two patients who have exactly the same diagnosis may respond quite differently from each other.

your own life. With a minor illness such as the flu, you may be emotionally irritable, lack physical energy, and not be able to carry out life's responsibilities for a few days. Even though you're back in the swing of things quickly, the illness still affects you. Have you ever missed something you really wanted to do but couldn't because you were sick and felt very disappointed? Has a test grade ever suffered because you were sick when trying to study for a test or while taking a test? The point is that everyone's performance is affected by sickness; thus, self-esteem is affected as well. You may be able to perform well enough to get by, but your performance will be less than optimal and can cause emotional distress.

DEPENDENCY: THE SICK ROLE

Once a person has been diagnosed as "sick" with a specific set of symptoms, she's excused from role responsibilities by society. Traditional North American cultural sick role beliefs assume that the sick person and family will seek out and cooperate fully with healthcare professionals, who are supposed to know more than the patient and family about the healthcare problem and how to correct it. It is assumed that the sick person wants to get well and will do everything as instructed by healthcare providers to get better as quickly as possible.[4]

This model implies a passive and compliant patient who trusts healthcare providers and who is motivated to get better and do whatever she's told in the manner in which she's told to do it. The healthcare provider is placed in a position of authority and dominance over the patient, and the patient has very little control over her situation. However, many patients and families emotionally object to the above-mentioned scenario of what they are "supposed" to do when they are ill.

Since the 1970s, feminist therapists have been promoting egalitarian relationships between healthcare professionals and patients instead of the more traditional view of the health professional as dominant and powerful and the patient as subordinate. Credited to the feminist movement has been the growing trend for a consumer orientation to relationships between patients and healthcare providers, with the patient viewed as a client and a partner in decisions about treating her health problem.[5]

For some people, the worst part of being sick is that they have to depend on others to take care of them. They can't stand the thought that they are no longer independent and productive and, at least temporarily, have to give up social, professional, and community roles that are important to their self-esteem. Some people try to keep going until they are extremely ill. They may be resentful, react with anger, and refuse to cooperate. They may feel powerless to control what is happening to them, and they may refuse to go along with the usual procedures.

For example, say that your patient just returned from surgery, is still recovering from the anesthetic, and is sedated. Yet he insists that he is getting up to go to the bathroom, *now*! After he refuses to use the urinal despite your encouragement, you decide to go and ask a colleague to help you get him up. As you return to the room with an assistant, you find him climbing over the side rail and have to run to catch him before he falls on the floor. He may have been thinking, "She doesn't know what she is talking about. Of course I can go to the bathroom by myself."

On the other end of the dependency continuum is the person who doesn't want to perform self-care activities for herself even after physically recovering to the point of being able to perform them. For example, the patient may use the call light and ask for assistance in going to the bathroom when she's physically able to be up and moving about on her own. Then, after you help her to the bathroom, she wants you to wash her completely and refuses to bathe herself even partially. This patient doesn't seem to want to give up the sick role; in fact, she may enjoy the attention she's receiving from healthcare professionals and others in her life. Some patients may retain the sick role because they want to avoid social commitments and work roles. Some patients may give up hope of ever resuming societal roles and may believe the only way to obtain respect and approval is through sickness. This attitude reflects low self-esteem.

In addition, some patients may also feel insecure and incapable of doing things on their own, even though they have recovered physically. For example, a patient who leaves the protective environment of a coronary care unit may feel insecure and fearful that if she performs too many self-care activities, she may bring on another heart attack.

The sick role involves cultural assumptions with many individual variations and reactions. These variations and reactions range from rejection of the dependent role and denial of behavioral changes needed to adapt to an altered health state, to submission to dependency and feelings of being incapable of returning to nonsick roles. Thus the sick role results in varied emotional responses based on the person's perception of the situation.

EMOTIONAL RESPONSES

Emotional reactions have been noted throughout the physical and psychosocial stages of illness and the sick role. Painful emotions always accompany physical and mental illness. Sadness, fear, and anger are prevalent during serious illness. However, admitting to emotional pain isn't socially acceptable to many North Americans, as well as to

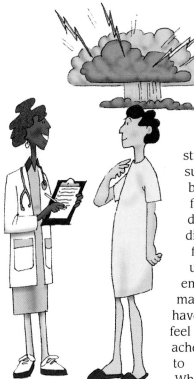

many other cultural groups. North Americans typically can admit physical pain within limits, but emotional pain may be considered a sign of weakness.

When emotions and tensions are held in, physical, emotional, and mental symptoms of stress arise because of the resulting release of stress chemicals.[6] The cartoon on this page suggests that repressed emotions lead to a blow-up. Without a release of emotions, feelings of sadness can progress to clinical depression, specific fears can progress to diffuse anxiety, and anger may be manifested as hostility and resentment. The figure on page 99 lists examples of physical, emotional and mental signs of stress that many of us have experienced.[7] For example, have you ever been so upset that you could feel tension in your muscles or gotten a headache? Have you ever felt irritable and unable to concentrate because you were upset? What did you do to relieve the emotional tension you felt? These same signs are present in patients and families who are reacting to the stresses associated with alterations in their state of health.

Repressed emotions can lead to blow-up.

EMOTIONAL RELEASE

How should you deal with your patients' emotions and your own emotions in healthcare settings? First, you must acknowledge and accept emotions. Don't pretend that emotions don't exist. Don't criticize emotions. Don't try to rationalize emotions or to change or fix them. Instead, allow emotions to be expressed because painful emotions want to be recognized. Encourage patients to ventilate their emotions. Patients or family members may yell and blame, placate and cry. Alternatively, they may be sarcastic and make jokes about their problems. After ventilation, they may be able to level with you and talk about their frustrations with their current situation.[8]

The emotions of sadness, fear, and anger in conjunction with typical behavioral responses to these emotions are found in the figure on page 100. The results of emotional expression include the healing of

EMOTION	(BECOMES)	RESULT
Sadness Fear Anger		Depression Anxiety Hostility/resentment

When emotions and tension are held within, signs of stress develop:

Physical Signs	Emotional Signs	Mental Signs
Hypertension	Irritability	Pessimism
Muscle tension	Exhaustion	Less concentration
Headaches	Boredom	Pickiness
Teeth grinding	Anxiety	Tunnel vision
Lower resistance	Depression	Mental errors
Colds	Withdrawal	Forgetfulness
Cold sores	Helplessness	Insomnia
Stomach acidity	Lethargy	
Stomach tightness		
Fatigue		

Physical, emotional, and mental signs of stress. (Adapted from Dugan, DO: Laughter and tears: Best medicine for stress. Nursing Forum 24:18, 1989. Reprinted with permission, Nursecom, Inc.)

sadness resulting from personal loss, the relief of fear, and the release of anger.

Everyone has built-in protective mechanisms that block painful emotions. These mechanisms are defenses that are activated automatically and unconsciously by the mind.[9] They're gradually lowered as the patient and family release emotions and adapt to their situation.[10] For example, sometimes a patient may deny that painful feelings exist, even though the person knows the truth at some level of awareness. Denial is taking place in a patient who learns in September that he has 3 months to live but who continues to plan his spring garden.

A patient found smoking in his room rationalizes that the hospital's rules are unfair and that he has a right to smoke if he wants. Actually, he may be feeling guilty. Of course he knows he shouldn't smoke, but he wants to save face by rationalizing. Sometimes a patient may feel one emotion but express the opposite emotion. A patient who is in pain smiles often and does what she is asked to do. In reality, she may be frightened and angry about her situation. She unconsciously wants to keep her anger controlled so that everyone likes her. So instead of showing anger, she smiles, which is the opposite of what she is feeling.

Emotion	Response	Results
Sadness	Sighing Tears Words	Healing
Fear	Shaking Perspiring Laughter Words	Relief
Anger	Ranting/ Raving Hitting Laughter Words	Release

Typical behavioral responses to sadness and anger. (Adapted from Dugan, DO: Laughter and tears: Best medicine for stress. Nursing Forum 24:18, 1989. Reprinted with permission, Nursecom, Inc.)

To be effective as a nurse, you must understand and accept the emotions of patients and families, no matter what, to create an atmosphere of safety and trust. Patients do the best they can, given their circumstances at that point in time. You need to develop a natural, spontaneous response to patients and families that conveys acceptance and interest in a genuinely nonjudgmental manner.

Understanding and acceptance do not mean that you have to agree with the patient. In the first example, you may not believe that the patient with cancer will be around to plant his spring garden, but you don't have to remove his hope by confronting him with the reality of death. An appropriate response is "I'll bet you've gotten a lot of enjoyment out of your gardens." Then see what he says next. Remember that he's doing what he can to manage the disease and collaborate with care, so nothing is wrong with denial. Some patients deny that they are dying until death itself occurs, and that's okay.

In the second example, you may not agree that the patient should smoke in the room—but you can find a place for him to smoke where it will be allowed, such as outside the building. In the third example, you recognize that the patient is really angry and in pain, yet she smiles. Give her pain medications to relieve the pain, and recognize that smiling is fine! Being understanding and accepting means that you make every attempt to listen attentively to the entire message, both verbal and nonverbal, and then communicate your understanding and acceptance back to the patient. Then you can take action based on your assessment and knowledge of what is really going on in the situation.

The Nurse's Emotions

Emotions can be contagious, and you may feel the same emotions and tensions that the patient and family feel. You may feel in danger of losing emotional control, and you may not know what to say or do. Acknowledge and accept emotions in yourself as well as your patient. Don' try to pretend that your emotions or your patients' emotions don't exist. They must not be ignored. They are present, real, and human.

To protect themselves from emotional pain, some nurses may pretend not to hear or see emotional responses. They might change the subject if patients start talking about something that's bothering them or change the subject without answering the question being asked. This nurse might also busy herself doing tasks, procedures, and paperwork, ignoring all painful emotions in herself and her patients and families. This nurse is using the classic Computer response to deal with her own feelings. She'll come across to the patient and family as uncaring, task oriented, and much too busy to be bothered. Withholding your own emotional response leaves the patient feeling out of control, unacceptable, and maybe even wondering if he's mentally unbalanced or crazy to feel the way he feels. You must carefully respond to the patient, both verbally and nonverbally, using the extremely important therapeutic communication technique of empathy.

Empathy versus Sympathy

The most important therapeutic communication technique to learn in dealing with the emotional responses of patients is to demonstrate empathy. When you demonstrate empathy, you participate in the life of another and perceive his or her thoughts or feelings. It means placing yourself in the patient's place and seeing the human side of the patient. It also means that you're sensitive to the patient's private world. Once you have perceived the emotional response, you must then respond to feelings and values in the situation and arrive at what is really important to the person. You must show you have sensitivity to the situation by communicating carefully with verbal and nonverbal skills to demonstrate that sensitivity. The result of empathy is that the person feels that he's really understood.[8,11]

Empathy also means that you remain emotionally separate from the other person, even though you can see the patient's viewpoint clearly. This is different from sympathy. Sympathy implies taking on the other's needs and problems as if they were your own and becoming emotionally involved to the point of losing your objectivity.[12] To empathize rather than sympathize, you must show feelings but not get caught up in feelings or overly identify with the patient's and family's concerns. You'll lose your objectivity if you share feelings so closely with a patient or family that your ability to think clearly and analyze problems becomes blocked.

When you are personally emotionally involved, you lose objectivity. For example, you as a nurse are overwhelmed with grief by the sudden death of your own father. You are too personally involved in this situation and feeling too much emotional pain to be therapeutic with members of your own family. That's why healthcare providers do not provide services to members of their own families. They're too personally involved and apt to lose objectivity. Their anxieties may be too high to think critically and effectively problem solve during the death or illness of a family member or close friend.

The Nurse as Advocator and Educator

The objective of using empathy is to convey interest in and understanding of the concerns behind painful emotions. You must listen long enough to allow the other person to experience release and ventilation. You function as a sounding board and personal confidant. Through the use of empathy, you must first convey to the patient that he is not alone and that you'll be there for him to help him through the situation. You'll act as a patient advocate to help the patient and family in doing whatever it takes to make sure their healthcare needs are met.[13]

Second, you should make it clear that there may be some things that the patient hasn't thought about that can be used to help handle the problem in a meaningful way. At this point, you become an educational resource helping the patient and family to think critically and analyze their situation. If a patient or family member can identify some areas that can be controlled, self-esteem will most likely increase and the underlying emotional distress will probably decrease.

In addition to practicing empathy, advocacy, and education, you can learn to use touch, humor, and tears to help patients express their emotions. These therapeutic techniques are the focus of upcoming chapters.

How to Facilitate Emotional Expression

Thus far, this text has presented therapeutic communication as it relates to the patient, family, and healthcare provider's general abilities to speak, see, hear, and comprehend messages. It has emphasized the uniqueness of each individual in perceiving, interpreting, and responding to messages based on past experiences. Also, recall that people who are under emotional strain will have more difficulty encoding and decoding messages. The next step is to focus on what you can say and do to make communication interactions therapeutic and to facilitate the expression of emotions—versus what you can say or do to block communication in the healthcare setting.

When you talk to a patient, you have a specific goal in mind. You may need to do an assessment, perform a treatment or procedure, or teach the patient or family member something about health. You need the patient's understanding and cooperation to attain your goal effectively and efficiently. During the interaction, you tune in to the nonverbal cues that signal emotional distress, the emotional tone of verbalizations, as well as the words that are spoken. You realize that you must manage emotional distress, if present, so that the patient can better understand and cooperate.

Let's assume that you're meeting a patient for the first time. You intend to do a screening health history, followed by a brief physical examination, and then you intend to teach the patient what he needs to know about a planned surgery. You're in an outpatient surgical center, your patient is 80 years old, and tomorrow she'll be having her cataracts removed. The patient is expected to go home when you are done and will return in the morning for the procedure. You are in a private, comfortable, and pleasant examination room. You have 30 minutes to get everything done before the next patient arrives.

You begin by introducing yourself, shaking the patient's hand, and offering her a comfortable chair. "Hello, I'm Sandy Baker, a student nurse. Please have a seat so we can begin." The patient sits down.

Next, you explain what you're going to be doing. "I'll be asking you some health questions and then I'll do a brief physical examination so we're sure that you're in good condition for surgery tomorrow. We'll also go over what you need to do tonight and what you'll be doing tomorrow when you return for your surgery. Did you have any questions about anything before we begin?"

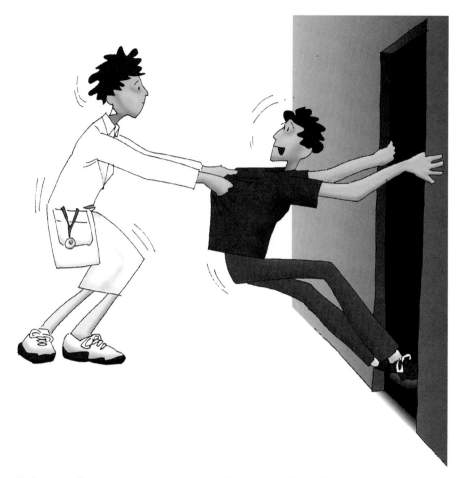

Patients can have major concerns about what you consider to be minor procedures.

Asking for any questions before beginning was a good thing to do. The student remembered to go to where the patient was, checking to see if she had any needs to be taken care of before beginning the interview. The patient replies, "I've never had any surgery in all my life. I hope it all turns out all right because I want to go back home and not be a burden to my children." Even though cataract surgery is a minor procedure and the prognosis is good, here is a patient who has some concern. This is typical. No matter what the procedure, even if it's minor, patients have emotional and psychosocial concerns. As depicted in the cartoon on this page, patients can have major concerns about what, to nurses, are minor procedures.

Blocks of Emotional Expression

In the previous scenario of the 80-year-old woman having surgery for cataracts, there are certain things you can say or do to facilitate or to block the expression of the patient's emotions and concerns. Blockers are presented first because they're used so commonly by nonprofessionals (and sometimes by professionals!) in an attempt to come to the emotional rescue of another person.[14]

CLAIMING THE PATIENT'S FEELINGS

It may be tempting, but don't use the phrase "I know how you feel" when listening to a patient's concerns. By saying, "I know how you feel," you are claiming the patient's feelings. That may make her angry. The patient may respond with, "How would you know! You don't look 80 years old and you are not a burden to your family!"

After all, how could anyone fully know the meaning of surgery and the emotions it produces for this patient or any other? You have never had the actual experience of being 80 and having surgery. The intent of the expression "I know how you feel" is valid because you want to show that you understand what the person is going through. But you can never know exactly how the person feels, so don't say it.

DISAPPROVAL

Another phrase to avoid is "You shouldn't feel that way." This phrase shows disapproval, and belittles and shames the patient. It also may be imposing your values on the patient or making a judgment about the patient. None of us can help the way we feel. We just experience the emotion. Everyone has the right to feel whatever emotion is present. You do not have to agree with what the patient says, but you must convey a willingness to hear the patient's viewpoint. Just listen openly to what the person has to say.

CHALLENGING OR DENYING STATEMENTS

"Why do you think you are a burden?" is an example of a question that is challenging and accusing and puts the patient on the defensive. Asking questions that start with *why* may cause resentment, insecurity, and mistrust. These are demanding questions that ask for rationalizations that the patient may not be able to give.

Likewise, don't deny a statement made by a patient about her feelings by saying something like, "I've met your family, and I'm sure that they don't think you are a burden." Instead, pursue the patient's reason for making the statement without using questions that begin with *why*. It's much better to ask questions that begin with *who*, *what*, *where*, *when*, or *how*. How to ask questions is discussed later in this chapter, under the section on facilitating communication.

FALSE REASSURANCE

You are giving false reassurance when you know things are not good and the prognosis is poor, but you say, "Keep your chin up, you're doing fine," "Everything will be fine," or "Every cloud has a silver lining." These clichés are attempts to pretend everything is fine and to cover up emotions. Nurses need to use reassurance to instill hope and to motivate patients, but false reassurance simply denies the patient's emotions and concerns.

There's nothing wrong with saying, "You're doing fine" when the patient really is doing fine. Follow up the statement with specific examples of where you see improvement. For example, if you find a normal blood pressure, you might say, "That's a good blood pressure." Alternatively, if you change a dressing, you might say, "That wound is healing nicely." But don't mislead the patient by giving false reassurance.

PEP TALKS

Typical examples of pep talks include use of expressions such as "Get hold of yourself" and "It's for your own good." Using these pep talks is a way to block emotions and get the patient to settle down. Again, however, the patient needs to express emotions. You'll need to be aware of the difference between offering encouragement, which every patient needs, and giving a pep talk, which will block the release of emotions.

GUILT

Don't make patients feel guilty about their emotions. Here's one avenue to avoid. Imagine that you're talking to a patient who's crying. In response, you say, "Think of your family. They're depending on you. You must be strong for them." This patient might be feeling very vulnerable and out of emotional control. Now, to top it off, she feels guilty!

Imagine another patient feeling sad about her physical condition. In response, you say to her, "Don't feel bad. Other people have it a lot worse than you do." Not only do these guilt-provoking responses not help, they hurt!

ADVICE

Don't give patients and families your advice. Advice means to give your opinion. For example, "You've got to think positive" is giving advice. In a related example, say a family is upset about what to do with grandma, who has a diagnosis of Alzheimer's disease. You say, "I think you should put your mother in a nursing home." You were trying to deal with their worries by making a decision and settling things for them. But when you give someone advice—your opinion—about what to do, you not only block emotional expression, but you take away the person's right to make the decision. You imply that you know what is best and how to take care of the emotional dilemma.

Instead of giving advice, first allow the family to express all their concerns, and then explain their options. Giving advice is much different than giving someone all the options and explaining all options. Once the options are known, the patient and family have the right to make the decision as to what's best for them. So instead of advice, allow emotional expression, then give options and discuss them. Stress that you're only giving options. For example, options would include "you could put your grandmother in a nursing home, you could take your grandmother home to live with you, or you could put her in adult day care while you work," and so on. Then you'd discuss the advantages and disadvantages of each option.

DEFENSIVENESS

Don't act defensively. Suppose a patient makes a negative comment about the care he is receiving either from you or a colleague. Instead of defending yourself or your colleague immediately, allow the patient to fully express the distrust and insecurities he feels, along with the specifics of the situation. Then give him information about the situation as you see it.

Remember that patients may place blame on someone else as a coping mechanism. Even so, this situation can be very difficult for you to handle, whether or not the patient has a legitimate complaint. It may be best to listen to the patient, being as open and nonjudgmental as you can, and then seek help from your clinical supervisor.

Facilitating Emotional Expression

Instead of blocking emotional expression and concerns, you need to learn how to facilitate self-acceptance and emotional release in your patients. You can do so through the use of nonverbal attentiveness and basic specific verbalizations to validate the meaning of the emotional content of the patient's message. Validation of the message is very important, because you must not only correctly perceive and interpret the patient's message but you must let the patient know that you have correctly understood what he has expressed to you. If you validate, then the chances of the patient recognizing that he has been understood will certainly increase.[8]

NONVERBAL ATTENTIVENESS

When you wish to be therapeutic and empathic, you need to listen very carefully and attentively.[15] First, sit down face to face, about 3 or 4 feet away from the person. You'll be best able to watch for nonverbal behaviors and pick up on them when sitting face to face. You have a much better chance of communicating clearly, of understanding what is being said, and of being understood by others. Lean forward, with a relaxed body posture. Look the person in the eyes as you talk to him. Nod your head and smile at appropriate intervals.

Sitting down on the same level with the person and looking at him as he speaks implies that you have time to relax and talk, and that you are not in a rush to be done and off to something else. If the patient feels relaxed and not rushed, he's more likely to freely converse and express emotions and concerns to you. In addition, when one person stands and the other sits during a conversation, the person sitting has less power than the person standing does. The patient is already in a dependent position because he can't meet his own healthcare needs. If you stand and the patient sits, the patient may feel even more dependent, with you as the authority figure. This may block his emotional expression.

Also, pull the curtain or close the door to give the patient privacy as you communicate. Patients will be more willing to talk confidentially and feel free to discuss emotions and concerns when they are in a private environment.

VERBAL FACILITATORS

You can use several basic verbal techniques to facilitate the expression of emotions and concerns. Most important, many verbal facilitators will validate the correct interpretation of the message for you and the patient, thus promoting understanding.[14]

General Leads

General leads encourage the patient to keep talking. They include such expressions as "please go on," "uh huh," and "yes."

Restatement

The purpose of restatement is to make sure of the implications of the words. You send feedback to the patient so he can be sure his message has been accurately received. The 80-year-old patient who is having cataract surgery says, "I don't want to be a burden to my family."

You would say in return, "It sounds like you're concerned that you won't be able to care for yourself after this surgery." Don't use the exact same words to reflect back to the patient. Doing so can be highly annoying, and makes you sound like a parrot if you say, "You don't want to be a burden to your family." The patient might respond with, "That's what I just said."

Clarifying and Focusing

You can also have the patient expand and focus on an issue by asking a question to assess the meaning of the message further. For example, "What do you think is going to happen with this surgery that will make you a burden to your family?"

Clarification is called for when there are many ways an idea could be interpreted. For example, the idea of "burden" is a rather abstract idea, and you need to get an indication of what that means to the patient. All clarification should be specific. The patient may respond, "My three children all want to take off work tomorrow to be with me for surgery. Then one of my daughters wants to stay overnight with me when she has her own family to take care of. They shouldn't have to worry about me." In addition, be sure to clarify dubious pronouns, such as "they" in this example. Clarify pronouns by asking, "Who are 'they'?"

Offering Information

Offer information after the patient has ventilated and expressed concerns, and when you believe that you have an accurate perception of the meaning of the situation for the patient. For example, to the 80-year-old surgical patient, you might say, "We need only one family member or friend here with you tomorrow for surgery. Everyone does not need to be here. You're scheduled to have surgery at 7:30 and should be discharged by noon. You'll need to go home and rest, but you should be able to stay by yourself at home." Give information appropriate to help the patient make decisions and plan, as well as information related to health teaching.

Asking Related Questions

Questions are useful for eliciting more information about a subject. You might want to ask, "Do you live alone?" to obtain more information about the patient's living situation. That information gives you a basis for negotiating realistic discharge plans with the patient. Sometimes questions can be closed-ended, requiring only a yes or no response. Other times, it may be more useful to ask an open-ended question that requires a wide-ranging answer. Examples start with "What do you think about. . . ," "What happens when you. . . ," and so on. Questions can also be used to obtain comparisons and a better understanding of the situation, such as "Is this different from your other experiences?" or "Perhaps it was like this?"

Stating Observations

A key part of the communication process is to watch the patient's nonverbal behavior. Say you go into a patient's room just as she slams a nightstand drawer. You ask, "What's going on?" The patient scowls at you and says, "Nothing." The nonverbal cues don't match the spoken words. You say, "Well, the look on your face and the slamming drawer suggests that you're angry about something." Always clarify conflicts between verbal and nonverbal cues, and remember that actions speak louder than words. Be very careful not to make an observational statement that claims the patient's feelings. For example, a statement like, "We certainly are upset, aren't we?" may only serve to infuriate the patient further.

Summarizing

At the end of a conversation, review the key ideas that were discussed. A summary validates the major points you intended to make. You could say something like, "Today we reviewed what will happen tomorrow before, during, and after surgery, and what you'll need to do after you're discharged." You could end with "Have I missed anything?" or "Do you have anything you'd like to ask, or add?" The patient can then add relevant information that was previously not addressed.

Managing Personal Emotions

You'll also have to learn to manage your own emotions effectively. Without successful self-management, nurses can become burned out. The burnout syndrome involves an emotional withdrawal that causes you either to leave your job or do as little as possible to get by. Painful feelings associated with burnout include fatigue, boredom, and frustration. The person with burnout becomes very negative and criticizes patients, colleagues, and self.[15,16]

To prevent burnout, you'll need to follow an exercise program and practice relaxation techniques. Maintain good nutritional practices, and get enough sleep. Do all the same things you tell patients to do for optimal health. You must take time to play and have fun, and you'll need to learn not to take your work home with you. It's very important to develop friends who are also colleagues who can be sounding boards for you and thus tremendous emotional support. Student nurses usually are very supportive of each other, and the attitude that "we're all in this together and will help each other" is critical to emotional survival even after school ends. Tips to prevent burnout are listed on page 112.[17,18]

In addition, nursing students must learn to control their nervousness in patient care situations. Remember, emotions are transmitted back and forth between people. You will be transmitting your anxieties to the patient, which will make the patient nervous. Even newborn babies, our tiniest patients, can sense anxiety in the person who is holding them and will respond by crying and struggling.

The first injection, the first dressing change, the first anything typically makes students nervous to the point of having worried facial expressions and shaking hands. Students fear making a mistake. It also makes many students nervous to have an instructor watch and evaluate the procedure. The patient senses the nervousness, and many patients actually provide encouragement and support to students because they recognize how nervous the students are.

If you are very nervous, there's no way that you can focus on the patient's emotions because all you can concentrate on is the procedure and your own feelings about it. As you become calm and confident in doing technical procedures, you will be better able to focus on the patient's emotional state. As comically shown in the cartoon on page 113, students feel many pressures. Please realize that it takes a lot of time, practice, and experience with patients to learn how to communicate effectively and therapeutically.

TEN BURNOUT

Prevention Tips

Stress is involved with the condition of living and cannot be avoided. You can, however, become more aware of the sources of stress and learn to prevent, adapt, or reduce the level of intensity. Many times it is not the stress that causes the trouble; it is the failure to perceive, copy, or adapt to the situation.

Ten tips on stress prevention, management, and reduction

1. Try to avoid taking on too much work as a persistent work style. Working hard is not the same as assuming tasks that you know cannot be completed successfully.

2. Try to avoid excesses in your lifestyle. Overeating, overdrinking, and overdieting lead to guilt or physical symptoms that, in turn, lead to stressful living.

3. Make yourself take a break at regular intervals to change the pace. Holidays and vacations should be constructive periods for self-improvement.

4. Pursue leisure time activities that completely take your mind off work problems or family problems. Activities that are considered to be thinking, feeling, and moving types are holistic in nature.

5. Avoid situations that persistently cause stress, if at all possible. Break habits that produce irritations.

6. Sleep is important, and by now you should know how much you need.

7. Cultivate an attitude of openness in discussing problems with family members, work colleagues, supervisors, subordinates, and so forth. Do not allow yourself to fall into the "silence syndrome."

8. Learn and practice methods of conscious relaxation. Make it a daily habit at a planned time. If necessary, join a class in yoga, transcendental meditation, or dance, or take part in sports or other physical activity.

9. Try to become a more perceptive person regarding yourself. How do you perceive yourself? Listen to your body and try to improve your body image, which is central to development of a positive self concept.

10. Take a good look at your lifestyle and make the changes that will bring you satisfaction and help you to become a "self-actualized" person.

Tips to prevent burnout.

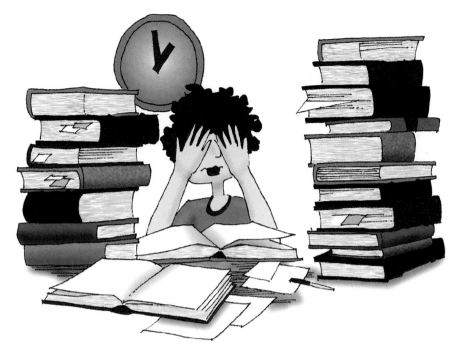

Nursing students feel many pressures.

SUMMARY

This chapter described emotional reactions to the stress of illness in the patient, family, and nurse. Therapeutic skills involving the use of empathy are essential to enable emotional expression. You must respond carefully to patients, considering what you are going to say and how you are going to say it. You need to determine what you'll be doing when you're speaking and where the conversation will take place. In addition, you must consider your role and relationship with the person with whom you'll be communicating. You must recognize that you can't be therapeutic when you are emotionally involved with a person, because objectivity is lost.

COMMUNICATION EXERCISES

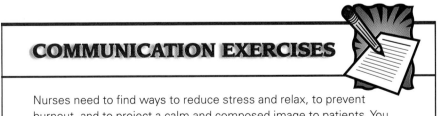

Nurses need to find ways to reduce stress and relax, to prevent burnout, and to project a calm and composed image to patients. You need to become aware of muscle tension and the need for relaxation.

These exercises are examples of popular relaxation techniques to help you reduce your stress level. You can use relaxation techniques when you're tense, for example, or before you perform a procedure for the first time. First, practice lying down either at home or in the nursing school laboratory, possibly with soft music of your choice playing in the background. With practice, you'll be able to relax almost anywhere and get results in a few minutes. This ability will become useful in clinical settings. You can also teach the techniques to patients to help them relax.

1 Progressive relaxation.[19] To do it, lie down and follow these steps.

- First, tighten the toes of both feet, and feel how the toes are in the tightened state. Now, let go and observe the feeling that accompanies release.

- Next, tighten your calves and thighs. Feel the tension, then let go and feel the sensation of relaxation.

- Then tighten your buttocks, hips, and abdominal muscles. Feel the tension, then let go and feel the sensation of relaxation.

- Now tighten the muscles of your chest and upper back. Feel the tension, then let go and feel the sensation of relaxation in this area.

- Tighten your hands and arms by making a fist and flexing your elbows. Feel the tension, then let go and feel the sensation of relaxation.

- Tighten your shoulders by raising them toward your ears. Feel the tension, then let go and feel the sensation of relaxation in this area.

- Now tighten your throat, neck, jaw, face, eyes, forehead, and scalp. Feel the tension, then relax each area and feel the sensation as the tension is released.

- Now raise and lower your eyebrows several times, then your eyebrows together in a frown. Then release the tension and feel the relaxation of the eyebrows.

- Finally, tighten all the muscles in your entire body, from toes to scalp. Hold it as long as you can. Then release the tension and become limp as a rag doll.

To finish the exercise, say to yourself, "I am relaxed, I am relaxed, I am relaxed." Check your body for any tense areas. If you find one, tell it to relax. Now lie quietly and enjoy your state of relaxation.

2 In an exercise called visual imagery, you'll picture yourself in the most beautiful, relaxing location you can envision.[20] Sitting on a beach in the warm sun, for example. Close your eyes and hear the waves splashing against the shore. Feel of the warm sun on your skin. Feel the warm ocean breeze on your face. See the gulls gliding gracefully across the glistening water. Say to yourself, "I am relaxed, I am relaxed, I am relaxed." Perhaps you prefer the mountains or a cool, shady spot. Just make sure the visual image has meaning to you. This is another good technique that can be used to help patients relax.

3 Practice using the basic communication techniques described in this chapter to demonstrate empathy toward a classmate. Use nonverbal attentive behaviors and verbal facilitation strategies to encourage a classmate to express his ideas and feelings about an important life event. For example, discuss taking care of a patient for the first time, a special birthday or anniversary, a championship sporting event, or something similar. Have one student tell the story of the important life event and the other use empathic communication techniques to listen fully and facilitate the expression of ideas and emotions. After the storyteller finishes, the listener should summarize her perception of the content and feelings expressed to validate the storyteller's message. The storyteller then states whether or not he thought the summary was accurate. If the summary is good, the listener has shown sensitivity to the other's private world using empathy. Understanding, and communication of that understanding, has been accomplished. You might even videotape these interactions and analyze empathic abilities by critiquing nonverbal attentive techniques, verbal blocks, and facilitators.

References

1. Festinger, LA: A Theory of Cognitive Dissonance. Stanford University Press, Stanford, California, 1957.
2. Martin, H, and Prange, A: The stages of illness: Psychosocial approach. Nursing Outlook *10*:168, 1962.
3. Kübler-Ross, E: On Death and Dying. Macmillan, New York, 1969.
4. Parsons, T: The Social System. Free Press, New York, 1951.
5. Enns, CZ: Feminist Theories and Feminist Psychotherapies: Origins, Themes, and Variations. Harrington Park Press, New York, 1997.
6. Selye, H: The Stress of Life. Mcgraw-Hill, New York, 1976.
7. Dugan, DO: Laughter and tears: Best medicine for stress. Nursing Forum *24*:18, 1989.

8. Rogers, CR: Client-Centered Therapy. Houghton Mifflin, New York, 1951.
9. Freud, S: Complete Psychological Works: Sigmund Freud. Hogarth Press, London, 1964.
10. Zook, R: Learning to use positive defense mechanisms. American Journal of Nursing 98:16B, 1998.
11. Sutherland, JA: Historical concept analysis of empathy. Issues in Mental Health Nursing 16:555, 1995.
12. Sundeen, SJ, et al: Nurse-Client Interaction: Implementing the Nursing Process, ed 5. Mosby, St. Louis, 1994.
13. Kozier, B, Erb, G, and Blais, K: Concepts and Issues in Nursing Practice, ed 2. Addison-Wesley, Redwood City, California, 1992.
14. Iveson-Iveson, J: The Art of Communication. Nursing Mirror 156(5):47, 1983.
15. Egan, G: The Skilled Helper: A Model for Systematic Helping and Interpersonal Relating, ed 2. Brooks/Cole, Monterey, California, 1982.
16. Freudenberger, H, and Richelson, G: Burnout: The High Cost of High Achievement. Bantam, New York, 1980.
17. Jaffe, D, and Scott, C: From Burnout to Balance. McGraw-Hill, New York, 1984.
18. Mazer, E: 10 Sure-fire stress releasers. Prevention 34:104, 1982.
19. Jacobson, E: Progressive Relaxation. University of Chicago Press, Chicago, 1938.
20. Samuels, M, and Samuels, N: Seeing with the Mind's Eye. Random House, New York, 1975.

CHAPTER 5

Breaking Through Barriers to Successful Communication

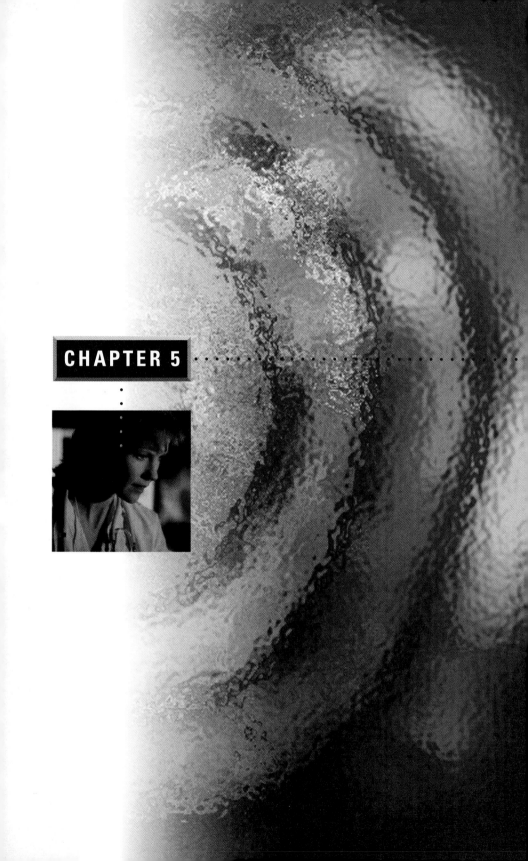

CHAPTER 5

Breaking Through Barriers to Successful Communication

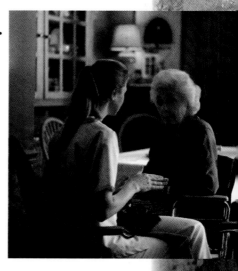

Chapter Objectives

AFTER READING THIS CHAPTER,
YOU WILL BE ABLE TO:

1. Summarize characteristics of responsive and assertive therapeutic communication strategies.

2. Describe how differences in patients' physical abilities, mental abilities, and desires to participate in care planning affect therapeutic communication.

3. Describe four basic communication patterns based on research by Bem and Wheeless.

4. Identify typical verbal and nonverbal reactions to stressful patient care situations for each of the basic communication patterns in objective 3.

5. Describe therapeutic communication strategies for patients or family members who are using aggressive or passive verbal and nonverbal communication behaviors as a means of coping.

THE PURPOSE OF THIS CHAPTER IS TO GO BEYOND BASIC THERAPEUTIC techniques and discuss therapeutic communication strategies for responding verbally and nonverbally to a patient or family member who is having trouble coping with health problems. For example, patients or family members may be angry, have difficulty expressing what they really think, or have difficulty making decisions. You can learn to choose your verbal and nonverbal communication behaviors carefully and formulate appropriate responses. Doing so will improve your therapeutic communication abilities.

The first step in breaking through communication barriers in stressful situations is to recognize that patients and family members erect behavioral barriers when they have a problem or their needs aren't being met. They're probably reacting to their own fear. Fears may be related to pain, lack of privacy, powerlessness, grief, any number of problems really, and the resulting inability to effectively cope with the situation. As described in Chapter 3, fears threaten self-esteem. As a result of these threats to self-esteem, people react. Expect a reaction. There will be one. Always keep in mind, however, that patients or family members are probably reacting to fear, not to you.

Sometimes, the behaviors of patients or family members become so intense that they upset you. For example, a patient may respond to you in an aggressive Blamer style or in a nonassertive and passive Placater style, as described by Satir.[1] You may feel anger toward the Blamer or feel exasperated with the Placater. You must learn to control your response.[2] In this chapter, these communication patterns of the Blamer and Placater will be expanded using additional theories and research by Bem, Dymer, Wheeless, and Dierks-Stewart.[3–5]

The focus of this chapter is on understanding aggressive and passive communication patterns commonly demonstrated by patients and families who are having difficulty coping. An emphasis is placed on therapeutic communication strategies that can be used to offset typical aggressive and passive communication patterns. The chapter concludes with examples of clinical problem situations that require therapeutic communication strategies of varying assertiveness and responsiveness.

Taking Control of Your Emotions

When you become upset, the fight-or-flight reaction, which has been described by Selye, occurs in your body.[6] The response is involuntary, so you need to become tuned in and aware of what your body is telling you. You will probably first feel tension. Although your first instinct might be to fight or to give in to a particular behavior a patient or family member is displaying—or perhaps you'd rather ignore the behavior that is upsetting to you—these responses on your part would not be therapeutic. First, break the tension you are feeling by taking some deep breaths, closing your eyes for a minute, speaking more slowly, getting a drink of water, or sitting down and leaning back. Laughter can also be used to release tension and will be the topic of Chapter 7.

You must also learn to recognize your typical style of behavior when you become upset, and you must learn to control these behaviors when you communicate therapeutically. Although the styles have been humorously categorized by Lachman, you may find one or more of the following categories that describes your typical response when you become upset.[2]

- *The volcano.* This person is also known as a hothead. He's quick to become upset, he blows up, and then he's done. He doesn't call names.

- *The tiger.* This person enjoys being upset and believes that she can say or do anything she wants. She may even call someone a name. Later, she expects to be forgiven because she says something like, "I'm sorry. I was angry when I said that."

- *The acorn collector.* This person doesn't like conflict and is slow to get upset. He collects grievances about a situation over a period of time and then will hurl them at someone when he has had enough. The acorn collector then will forgive and forget about the problems.

- *The grudgesaver.* This person also doesn't like conflict and is slow to become upset. However, the grudgesaver doesn't forgive and forget, and he has a hard time getting over an outburst directed at him.

After you identify your typical style or styles of behavior when you are upset, you must compare your typical behavior with what it means to respond assertively and level with the person whose behavior is upsetting you. Assertiveness and leveling are only possible when you have strong self-esteem and when you believe that you can control your behaviors and perform specific actions and behaviors that will affect your relationships with others. Throughout this book, assertiveness and leveling are used interchangeably. As noted in Chapter 3, the word leveling is Satir's term for acting in an assertive manner.[1]

Assertiveness and leveling behaviors are based on the assumptions that all people have rights to the things they need in life and that behaviors that violate those rights are not acceptable. This assumption applies to both you and your patient. You have rights that must be upheld, and your patient has rights that must be upheld. Understanding the rights of nurse, patients, and families is fundamental to becoming an assertive nurse. Assertive nurses know how to level, that is, to speak what is on their minds effectively to defend their personal rights and the rights of patients in their care.

Assertiveness in Nursing Practice

Lack of assertiveness plagued the nursing profession for many years for two reasons. First, nurses used to be socialized to be submissive to physicians and nurse supervisors through nursing education programs. Second, throughout most of the history of professional nursing, nurses have been primarily women. In many instances, women have been traditionally socialized into a more passive role.[7,8]

The women's movement during the 1970s brought about an interest in assertiveness as a special skill for women in general. Change has been slow in coming, but many nurses are now taking a more active and assertive role in the care of patients.[7,8] Also, a growing number of men now are enrolled in nursing programs and are professional nurses. Assertive communication techniques are taught in nursing education programs.

No one is born assertive. Assertiveness is a learned behavior. One advantage you have in working with patients in a professional role is that, usually, patients don't know you personally. As you practice assertiveness in nursing clinical situations, you may find it much easier to be assertive with people you don't know. Once you have a role established, such as wife, husband, mother, father, daughter, or son, the behavioral styles are ingrained and are much harder to change. You're expected to act in certain ways, verbally and nonverbally, in your known role. Established patterns in relationships that have evolved over many years are very difficult to change. When acting as a nurse, you may need to be more or less assertive than you would in some other roles you already have, such as the role of spouse.

You must also recognize that everyone communicates with different degrees of assertiveness depending on the circumstances. How do you respond to a close friend who is angry? How do you respond to your mother and father when they give unsolicited advice on what you should do about a situation? How do you respond to a nursing professor who is criticizing your clinical performance? How do you respond to the insistent telephone salesperson who calls and, no matter what you say, keeps trying to sell you a product? How do you respond to a waiter who brought you cold food? The degree of assertiveness you use probably depends on the situation.

Patients come from highly varied backgrounds and are affected by their environment and the roles they play in each situation within that environment. You must recognize that people won't always respond in the same manner, even though the situation appears similar. Patients have learned different and preferred verbal and nonverbal behavioral responses to their environments. Many times, patients may respond in ways that may surprise you because the way they have learned to respond is so different from the way you have learned to respond to a similar situation.

Patient Participation in Care

The behavior of patients reflects the role that they're playing at any given point in time. In the patient role, the person may act more passively than they would under other circumstances, such as at work. There may be times when the patient is passive and unable to participate in goals and plans because of physical problems. For example, a patient having a heart attack needs immediate treatment and typically remains passive as these treatments take place. Any unconscious patient is entirely passively dependent on healthcare providers.

Highly anxious patients need much guidance and support from healthcare providers, and they may have a limited ability to think clearly. They may also have ineffective styles of communication. In these situations, the healthcare providers are probably making most of the decisions on behalf of the patient.

In many chronic, stable conditions, the healthcare provider and patient may be able to develop a partnership relationship, depending on patient and family preferences and the communication skills of the healthcare provider.[9] Patients may have preferences for how active they want to be in the management of their care. However, don't assume that all patients want to be full partners in all aspects of their care, even though they are mentally and physically capable of it. Some patients would prefer to leave everything up to healthcare providers. A typical statement by such a patient might be, "I don't want to know the details. Just fix it!"

Although this is true of some patients, however, it isn't true of most. It has been reported that healthcare providers often underestimate the extent to which patients want to know about alternatives.[10] Patients may hesitate to voice their questions and concerns. Many feel that they don't want to be any trouble to anyone. Some may add the statement, "Just tell me what I'm supposed to do." These passive patients may believe they are being so-called good patients, whereas those who ask questions and have different ideas than the healthcare provider may view themselves as uncooperative "problem" patients.[10]

Many patients have unique perceptions and ideas about the nature of a health problem and its consequences. For some patients, personal values and beliefs that are different from yours will guide the treatments they choose to accept or refuse. As depicted in the cartoon below, patients are sometimes treated with a clinically objective approach to pathophysiology and the disease, with minimal attention given to the patient's subjective experience. An important goal of nursing care is to encourage patients to speak openly and state their values, beliefs, and expectations regarding their health problem. Try to determine how *the patient* wants the problem to be treated and resolved.

Although people behave in many different ways depending on the situation they're placed in, everyone tends to behave and respond in ways that feel most comfortable, according to how they have learned to communicate under stress. If you can recognize and understand

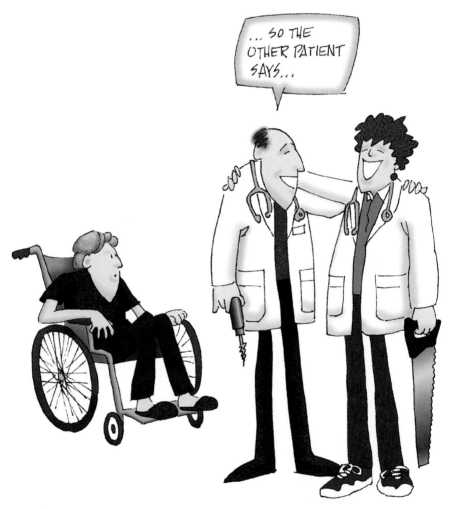

Sometimes patients are treated with little regard for their subjective experience.

typical communication patterns in yourself and your patients, you can learn to control your customary responses and to respond with versatility in your therapeutic communications. Versatility as a communicator implies flexibility with what's happening in the situation.[6] You need to be a very versatile communicator to develop mutually acceptable health-specific goals and work toward them effectively and efficiently with a wide variety of patients. This takes much practice. It is not an easy thing to do.

The Versatile Therapeutic Communicator

Two important dimensions of personality—assertiveness and responsiveness—indicate versatility and competence in communication. The seminal research of Bem, Wheeless, and Dierks-Stewart has demonstrated that people tend to display different degrees of assertiveness and responsiveness.[3,5] However, each person has developed preferred assertive and responsive styles of communication that they usually display most of the time.

The most competent and versatile communicators are both highly assertive and highly responsive to other people in their typical style of communication.[11] But how much of each ingredient is needed? You need to develop the ability to modify the amounts of assertiveness and responsiveness you use depending on the behaviors of the person you are interacting with, as well as the demands of the situation.

ASSERTIVENESS

The main components of assertive behavior include the ability to tell others what you would like them to do, to refuse to do those things you don't want to do, to express positive and negative feelings, and to start, continue, and stop conversations.[12] In addition, all of these activities must be accomplished with respect for the personal rights of others. Assertiveness has been related to the need to be directive. The more assertive people are, the more they typically like to direct others, and they probably feel comfortable telling others what to do. Assertive people find it rewarding and satisfying to direct other people. Thus, they have a need to direct others because it makes them feel good.

Typical descriptive characteristics of a person who is considered assertive include

- ability to act as a leader
- strong personality

- forceful and dominant
- independent
- willing to take a stand
- able to defend one's beliefs.[11]

These characteristics are typically assigned to stereotypically masculine forms of behavior. However, many women also exhibit these behaviors. As noted in Chapter 2, it is important to avoid stereotyping individuals based on gender.

In contrast, nonassertive people find it much more difficult to direct others, and they're typically more submissive to others. Nonassertive people tend to feel uncomfortable telling others what to do, and they feel much better asking others to do something. Or they may hesitate to ask for help at all. Nonassertive people may prefer just doing the job themselves because it feels so uncomfortable to tell someone else what to do to help. They have difficulty saying what they think, and although they may not agree with what they're told to do, they do as they're told without objection to avoid rocking the boat or causing trouble by expressing what they really think. Thus, the term *passive* has been applied to the behavior of nonassertive people.

RESPONSIVENESS

Responsiveness involves the ability to be sensitive to the needs and wants of others. Responsive individuals are people oriented, are good listeners, and strive to make others feel comfortable during a conversation.[11] Responsive people typically enjoy the company of others.

Typical descriptive characteristics of responsive people include

- sensitivity to the needs of others
- attentive listener
- desire to make others feel at ease.

These people typically show their emotions. They usually enjoy being around people and helping people. They like the process of getting things done, and they like working with other people. These are qualities assigned to stereotypically feminine forms of behavior. Of course, many men also exhibit these behaviors.

In contrast to having responsive tendencies to others, nonresponsive people tend to be more task oriented than people oriented. They need to get things done and may prefer not to socialize because socializing takes time away from the task at hand. Showing emotions may be considered a sign of weakness.

Everyone exhibits some combination of assertiveness and responsiveness. The various blends of assertive and responsive communica-

tion competence patterns have been depicted as intersecting continu-
ums shown in the graph below. The combination of both the ability to
be assertive plus the ability to be responsive results in four possible
communication patterns.[3,5] These patterns can be categorized as
highly assertive and highly responsive (quadrant 1), highly assertive
and nonresponsive (quadrant 2), nonassertive and highly responsive
(quadrant 3), or nonassertive and nonresponsive (quadrant 4). To become a competent therapeutic communicator, you need to work on
becoming highly assertive and highly responsive to others. Your ability
to be assertive and responsive will change as you experience varied
patient and family encounters in your clinical practice. A primary goal
of nursing educators is to teach students to perform both of these
communication skills well. A self-assessment to rate your current levels of assertiveness and responsiveness is found in the communication exercises at the end of the chapter.

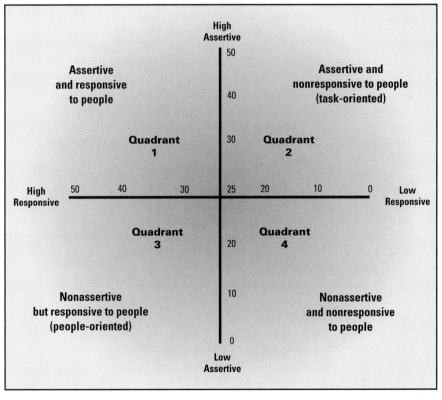

*Blends of assertive and responsive communication competence patterns. (Reprinted by
permission of Waveland Press, Inc. from McCroskey, JC and Richmond, VP:
Fundamentals of Human Communication. Waveland Press, Prospect Heights, Illinois,
1996. All rights reserved. Redrawn.)*

The most important point to keep in mind as you are interacting in a therapeutically assertive and responsive manner is the fact that you have rights, that the other person with whom you speak has rights, and that neither of you should have your rights violated. By recognizing and understanding typically assertive and responsive patterns in yourself and others, you will have a knowledge base for developing therapeutic communication strategies that include purposeful variation of the degree of assertiveness and responsiveness you use in each patient care situation. Each pattern of communication is described in the following sections for each of the four quadrants in the figure on page 127.[11] Implications for the types of communication patterns that may be manifested when people in each grouping are placed in stressful health care situations are also described. Nursing therapeutic communication strategies to be used when faced with these typical communication patterns are included in examples in the last section of this chapter.

Quadrant 1

People in quadrant 1 have highly assertive and highly responsive tendencies. Typically, they're persuasive and inspiring. They are open, outgoing, and self-confident. They have highly developed social skills and are spontaneous without being impulsive. They need adventure and excitement. They're competitive and like to take risks. These people enjoy attention and recognition. Typical occupations that require this type of personality include public speakers, salespeople, public relations personnel, and supervisors.

Given the above-mentioned description, you'll understand that these people may rapidly become impatient when they have to wait for something to be done. They don't like indecision, and they don't like a lack of enthusiasm. They get bored when things are too conventional. They want to be respected by others and work well with people. They like being in charge and telling others what to do to get goals and objectives accomplished.

Picture this person in any situation in which she feels threatened and out of control. For example, imagine that this person has just been hospitalized with a disease that will require many changes in lifestyle but is not yet being managed adequately. How might this person act as a patient? She may be pushy and overbearing. She may intimidate and manipulate. She could be restless and impatient. She may tend to be abrasively sarcastic, and she may lash out at whoever is nearby. When people who are highly assertive and highly responsive lose their temper, they tend to blow up and throw a tantrum.[4] The tendency is for this person to act in an aggressive manner and to use sarcasm.

Quadrant 2

People in quadrant 2 have highly assertive and nonresponsive tendencies. They work at a fast pace and tend to be goal oriented. Winning is more important than anything or anyone else. They like to be challenged and are easily bored. They are very direct about telling others what to do, and they expect people to be loyal and to follow all the rules. They have traditional values and ways of thinking. They need to be in authority, and they need to master and control every situation. Getting things done is very important, and they accept the responsibility for things to be done right. They are self-determined and ambitious. These people are dependable, organized, practical, and economical. Their typical occupations include chief executive officers of companies. Many physicians could be placed in this category.

These people do not like uncertainty. They cannot tolerate laziness because laziness means the job is not getting done. They are highly competitive. Getting the task done and winning is a higher priority than being responsive to the needs of others. They need to tell others what to do, and they dislike following someone else's lead. Showing emotions gets in the way of accomplishing the tasks at hand. Because they are traditional, disrespectful behavior is not appreciated. They do not like estimates, so when you approach such a person, know what you're talking about. These people like to be right. If they've made a mistake, an indirect approach is best. Don't tell them they're wrong. Instead, gently try to help them understand other perspectives on a situation.

When these people are stressed by illness and become upset with a problem situation, they may become extremely critical of whomever and whatever is standing in the way of accomplishing tasks how and when they want them done. These people tend to attack directly with open hostility, and they may complain loudly on and on about something that is bothering them. A wall goes up around them, and they may appear to be insensitive, distant, and unapproachable. They permit themselves to get angry and upset, but expression of feelings such as sadness, fear, or any other emotion that shows vulnerability isn't acceptable to them. They can be extremely stubborn, dogmatic, and rigid in how they think and act.[4] Thus, these people can become very aggressive, similar to patients in quadrant 1 but more openly hostile.

Quadrant 3

People in quadrant 3 have nonassertive and highly responsive tendencies. Their chief motivation is the need to be loved. These people are team oriented and want to keep the peace. They need to keep everyone happy. They are sociable and friendly, and they know how to listen actively. They are caring and devoted, trusting, and sensitive to the needs of others. They like helping others and are very kind. They like feeling emotional closeness with others and want to be popular with everyone. Instead of being directive, they will ask others to do things. They don't like to tell others what to do. Typical careers these individuals select involve service to others, such as transportation services and health service workers. Many student nurses at least begin nursing with this basic communication style.

These people don't like insensitivity and insincerity. They feel uncomfortable with disagreement. Self-centered, egotistical behavior is also not acceptable. They feel more comfortable following rather than leading other people because following results in less conflict in relationships.

Nonassertive and highly responsive may become very vulnerable and indecisive people during the stress of illness. They will attempt to suppress their anger and smile. They may become emotional, and they may be subjective and impractical. They are too other oriented, and they want to keep everyone happy. Keeping everyone happy also leads to difficulty in saying no to others and the tendency to be too agreeable.[4] These people may procrastinate because of their difficulty making decisions. Therefore, these people may become very passive and not want to discuss what upsets them about their care.

Quadrant 4

People in quadrant 4 have nonassertive and nonresponsive tendencies. They tend to have very high standards, and they're meticulous, exacting, and thorough. They like obtaining copious information and pay attention to every detail. They like perfection. They are logical and focused on outcomes. They appear reserved and calm, and they don't express emotions. They don't like taking risks, they're practical, they're most comfortable with consistency and routines, and they don't like change. These people are task oriented, and they're socially shy and withdrawn from others. They prefer to work alone, autonomously, because that way they can be sure everything will get done correctly. They may be slow to get things done because everything must be perfect. Typical occupations suitable to this personality include data processor, architect, engineer, and accountant.

These people don't like others who are arrogant or artificially sincere, nor do they like people who are careless or overly assertive. They like to be right, and they feel more comfortable following rather than leading others.

Under the stress of illness or problem situations, these people are highly analytical but may be incapable of making decisions and dealing with problems. They know what's right and what's wrong, and they may complain endlessly to everyone around them. However, they don't have the energy or social skills to deal directly with problem people or situations. They can talk negatively and at length about how everything is awful, acting gloomy and depressed about something disturbing them.[4] Because of their lack of social skills and limited ability to make decisions, these people are characteristically passive in relationships with healthcare providers.

Communication Difficulties

Most of the problems nursing students have in communicating therapeutically stem from a lack of understanding of typical communication patterns and ways that people are likely to react in stressful situations, such as during an illness. An inability to communicate assertively and responsively lies at the root of the communication difficulties. You need to know how to establish rapport and trusting relationships with patients who display different degrees of assertiveness and responsiveness, as well as to respond to situational circumstances affecting the pattern of communication.

When people are upset, their self-esteem is threatened, and they perceive that they are under attack. They will react. Typically, they either withdraw and are passive and submissive or they fight and become aggressive. People in quadrants 1 and 2 tend to become aggressive, showing hostility and sarcasm under stress. People in quadrants 3 and 4 tend to become passive in stressful situations. They may be too agreeable, tend to procrastinate, and whine or complain. Because of these differences in response, you need to become aware of how to respond to patients with each tendency.

How to Respond to Aggression

Assertiveness without regard for the rights of others is termed aggression. Aggressive people may demand that things be done their way. Others feel pushed to comply with these demands, even though it goes against their own feelings, rights, and needs. Thus, aggressive behavior is resented and often results in the alienation of others. You may encounter aggression either as open hostility or as the less obvious sarcasm.

OPEN HOSTILITY

Typically, the aggressive person is probably expecting you to fight with them or to give in to them. An irate patient is comically shown in the cartoon below. Instead, don't do either. Communicate therapeutically in an assertive and responsive manner.

First, let the patient express her emotions and blow off some steam while you listen carefully. Don't get upset in return. Take a deep breath and count to 10, which gets some oxygen flowing to your brain to help you think. You may need to do some positive self-talk, such as "I can handle this; I am strong; I can deal with this."

Typically, openly aggressive behavior is characterized by loud, angry words and blaming messages that start with *you*. Don't aggravate the person and attack her in return with *you* messages. For example, don't say, "How dare you speak to me that way!" Also, avoid other inflammatory statements that will only fuel the patient's fire, such as "You must be crazy!" or "How could you possibly think that!" Be careful not to find fault with who people are. It's the behavior that's the

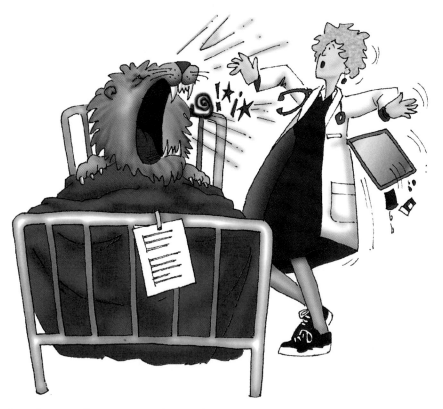

Sometimes you'll encounter an irate patient.

problem, not the person, so you must get to the reason for the behavior. Always try to describe situations and behaviors in a nonblaming manner.

First, you need to get the person's attention. If your patient is in the middle of a rage, she isn't thinking and she isn't hearing. You may need to interrupt the person by calling her name and saying, "Ma'am, Ma'am" until you have her attention for a moment. Sometimes you may need to make a noise; for example, drop a pen or a chart just to get her to stop for a moment and look to see what happened. Don't slam down a chart or pen, which could be interpreted as anger and aggression from you. Drop it on purpose, but make it look like it slipped out of your hand, just with the intent of making a noise. Once the patient hesitates, slip in your message, "I'd like to help you. Let's go sit down in the conference room and talk." Speak slowly, calmly, and quietly, using slow gestures. If you slow down, she will too.

Now, take the person to a private place and have her sit down, if you can. Sitting is a less aggressive position. You may need to stand up slowly if you were sitting when first approached by the aggressive person, and then ask her to sit down very calmly. Don't make any abrupt movements. If she refuses to sit down, you need to remain standing as well.

Listen attentively as she explains her problem, and send back to her what she's telling you using basic communication techniques, such as restatement and empathy. Listen for what she wants that will calm her down. Question her without antagonizing her, using an indirect approach. Be persistent to get down to the root of the problem. Speak from your point of view as you present what you see as going on in reality. Show that you're sincere in your desire to talk with her and help her solve the problem. Be sure to validate with her what you think the problem is.[4] Consider this scenario as an example.

> PATIENT'S HUSBAND: "I'm calling my lawyer! My wife hasn't gotten any @#$% help since she got here. You're not even feeding her! This is the worst hospital I've ever been in, bar none. You people have no idea what you're doing around here. . . ."

> STUDENT NURSE, INTERRUPTING: "Sir, I'd like to help you. . . ."

> PATIENT'S HUSBAND, INTERRUPTING: "I said I'm calling my lawyer. No one listens to anything around here. . . ."

> STUDENT NURSE: "Sir, I'd like to help you. Please come with me to the conference room so we can talk."

> STUDENT NURSE, NOW IN THE CONFERENCE ROOM WITH THE PATIENT'S HUSBAND: "Please sit down so we can talk. I heard you say that

your wife has a problem getting food. Can you tell me specifically what is going on?"

PATIENT'S HUSBAND: "My wife has cancer and she needs to eat to keep up her strength. She's starving in here! She didn't even get breakfast."

STUDENT NURSE: "Your wife was supposed to have special blood tests done this morning. As soon as they're completed, I'll see to it that she gets a tray right away. *(explaining reality)* I can see that you're very concerned about the care your wife is getting and that you want to make sure everything goes smoothly." *(using empathy)*

PATIENT'S HUSBAND: "We've been married for 30 years and she's never been sick. I want to do everything possible to beat this cancer."

STUDENT NURSE: "Good nutrition *is* very important to help her feel better. Let me check with the lab right away. I'll let you know what I find out about when she can eat. As soon as she can, I'll bring her something from our unit kitchen as a snack until her tray gets here. I'll be down to her room in 5 minutes to let you know what's going on."

SARCASM

Sarcasm is a less obvious form of aggression. The people-oriented responsive person tends to use sarcasm to disguise aggression. Sarcasm comes in the form of insults, snide remarks, or cynical comments. The person using sarcasm is termed passive aggressive. Sarcasm is aggressive because it has no regard for the feelings of others. The person using sarcasm may consider it socially unacceptable to be openly aggressive, hostile, or angry. Instead, the hostility comes out in nasty comments, either to anyone who will listen or directly to the person causing the problem.

The person using sarcasm expects the target person either to be hurt by the comment (flight) or to become upset and blow up (fight). Again, don't do either. Bring the sarcastic comment out into the open by asking questions in an assertive, calm, and quiet manner, "Was there something in that remark you just made?" This will need to be said in front of other people. The person making snide comments usually does so in front of others, counting on the fact that you will not make a scene in front of everyone. After you confront him, he may be able to tell you directly what's bothering him, and you can have a discussion of the problem. You should seek a private room for that discussion.

Sometimes bringing the comment to light will precipitate an outburst of openly aggressive behavior. The person may answer you with, "What's the matter? Can't you understand English?" You need to respond calmly, slowly, and with an even tone of voice, "I don't know what you meant by that comment. Please explain it to me." The person may then get angry and blow up. If so, proceed as described earlier by allowing them to blow off steam, interrupting him if necessary, and then listening carefully to discern the real issues. Then deal with the real issues. Show your sincerity and desire to talk, and get to the bottom of the situation.[4] Here's an example of an interaction with a sarcastic person.

> STUDENT NURSE, ENTERING THE ROOM: "Hi, Mr. Jones. This morning you need to be up in the hall and walking. When would you like to take a walk?"

> PATIENT, HOLDING HIS INCISION AND WINCING: "You must have left your brains at home when you came in this morning." *The patient in the other bed laughs.*

> STUDENT NURSE, IN A CALM AND MATTER-OF-FACT MANNER (ASSERTIVELY): "I don't appreciate that remark. I'd really like to help; what's the matter?"

> PATIENT: "Can't you take a joke? You're too sensitive."

> STUDENT NURSE, CALMLY, SLOWLY, AND QUIETLY: "I think there is a problem here. What's the matter? I'd like to help if I can."

> PATIENT: "You think I can just jump out of this bed, or what? Don't you know I had surgery yesterday and I'm in pain! I need a pain shot and sleep, not a walk."

> STUDENT NURSE: "I should have asked you how your pain was before I asked when you wanted to walk. Of course I'll get your pain medication. I have to be sure your blood pressure and pulse are okay first, then I'll go get the injection. I'll go as fast as I can."

> PATIENT: "Please hurry. I'm sorry I made that nasty comment. I just hate being stuck in bed like this."

When a patient is aggressive, it is important to realize that the anger and hostility are coming from within. At that point, you have to choose whether to respond with aggression, passivity, or assertiveness. Most of the time, what the person needs to settle them down has nothing to do with you personally. The person simply has a different perception of the situation than you do, and he isn't handling the situation well. You must get to the bottom of the problem to discover what's really bothering him and making him angry.

Don't react defensively to a personal attack. Avoid the accusation-defense-reaccusation cycle.[4] This cycle occurs when the patient says, "It's your fault that my wife didn't get her tray." You respond with, "It's not my fault." Then the person says, "It is, too, your fault. You're a nurse aren't you?" Nothing gets solved in this scenario. Instead, focus on the problem and ignore the accusation. Say something like, "I was not aware that there was a problem with her tray. Could you tell me what happened, please?"

Always remember that there's a reason patients or family members are acting the way they are. They're doing the best they can, but they may not be communicating effectively. If you make a mistake, such as the student in the second example who should have assessed for pain before asking the patient to walk, just admit it and try to rectify the problem. Everyone, including a nurse, has the right to make mistakes.

How to Respond to Passivity

A passive person may be too agreeable, may procrastinate, or may complain. In each case, therapeutic communication techniques can help you improve your interactions with the passive person.

TOO AGREEABLE

Many passive people have a hard time saying "no." They feel guilty if they say "no," and they don't want anyone to become angry with them or think poorly of them. They say "yes" and then get themselves in the bind of not being able to do everything they've committed to do. Then they can't do anything well because they have too much to do. They say "yes" to everything, even at high cost to themselves. They give in to others without protecting their own rights. If you're dealing with a people-oriented passive person, she doesn't want to offend you by saying "no" because she needs you to like her. It may get very frustrating dealing with this person when nothing gets done as she told you it would be.

Always, first show your concern and interest in a person who has a responsive pattern of communication. Ask how things are going, and inquire about family members. Then talk about the goals and objectives that need to be accomplished. As you talk about goals and objectives, make being honest as nonthreatening as possible. For example, say something like "I would appreciate it, if you have other things to do, if you'd tell me that you can't do what I'm asking." Watch out for unrealistic commitments by asking how the person plans to accomplish the activity. What you are asking may be impossible based on other commitments, or the person may simply not know what to do.[4] Here's an example.

A student nurse in home health was teaching a patient to give herself insulin injections. The student had given the patient reading material and a movie on self-injection that was to be completed by their appointment at 8 o'clock the next morning. When the student arrived at 8 am, the patient was flustered and said she had started to read but had to do laundry, pick up the children at school, make dinner, and then help the children with homework, and she didn't get to bed until late. In this situation, the student nurse needs to bring issues out into the open and help the patient define the problems.

> PATIENT: "I wanted to do everything, and I'm going to get to it today. I'm spread too thin, I think, and I'm having trouble getting things done. I'm sorry I'm wasting your time here. I know I need to learn how to do these injections myself. I've always taken care of my family. They come before anything."

> STUDENT NURSE: "You have many family responsibilities. I would really appreciate it if you would tell me when you don't think you'll be able to get something done. Believe me, I'll understand if you have other things to do. I know there are only so many hours in a day. What if I watch the movie with you and go over the most important points, then you can review these important points before we meet again?"

The student nurse has realized that asking the patient to read and watch a movie was too much and has come up with a compromise. The nurse needed to take a more active role in teaching the patient the material, and the patient agreed to review on her own, a more realistic plan for learning the techniques.

PROCRASTINATION

In addition, passive and responsive people may be procrastinators. They don't want to offend anyone, so they have difficulty making a decision. They get caught up in the emotions of the decision and can't see the logic of a choice. They want to smooth over problems, and they often let others make decisions for them. Such a person will give in and back down to avoid confrontation. The problem and issues need to be brought out into the open. You need to help the procrastinator define his problems, help him be realistic about what is going on, and then help him problem solve. Then you may need to coach him and meet with him on a regular basis to check his progress. This person needs guidance and someone to direct him.[4]

Say, for example, that a patient is trying to decide which nutrition class to attend to learn about a heart-healthy diet. He doesn't know which to attend. In one class, he knows the instructor from his church social group. In the other class, he has a personal friend. Instead of picking a class, he's worried about offending the friend or the instructor by not going to their class. Consequently, he hasn't signed up for anything. His emotions are blocking making a decision. He needs help in developing some form of people-oriented compromise. For example, what if he attends the class with the instructor he knows, then goes out to lunch with the friend, who can help him pick items that fit the diet from the restaurant's menu? You can also help him take into consideration the time classes are offered and total program costs. Problem-solving strategies are discussed in an upcoming chapter.

COMPLAINING

A passive person who is task oriented may be inclined to complain at length to anyone who will listen but may not have the energy or social skills to talk to the person who's the source of the complaints. This passive person may be looking for someone to act on her behalf and to solve the problem for her. Most important, listen closely, and let her feel important. This person is highly analytic, and she knows what's right and wrong. She keeps going over and over the same things and can be extremely negative. She tends to speak in generalities, so you'll need to ask her to be specific. *Who*, *what*, *when*, and *where* questions are appropriate. Once you know the specifics, state the facts as you see them and state your perception of the situation.[4] Here's an example.

PATIENT, IN A WHINING VOICE: "These things always happen to me. Nothing ever goes my way. I'm never getting out of here."

STUDENT NURSE: "What's wrong?"

PATIENT: "Everything is wrong, nothing is right."

STUDENT NURSE: "What happened, specifically?"

PATIENT: "It's the doctor. He was just here."

STUDENT NURSE: "What did he say to you?"

PATIENT: "He wants to run more tests, and I can't leave here."

STUDENT NURSE: "That's disappointing that you can't go home (empathy). Which tests does he want to run?"

PATIENT: "He wants me to have a stress test, and I want to get out of here."

STUDENT NURSE: "Did you talk with him about having it done on an outpatient basis?"

PATIENT: "No, he'd never agree to it."

STUDENT NURSE: "Well, to you it seems like this is a hopeless situation, and to me it seems we should inquire about having the test done as an outpatient procedure. If the doctor says no, what's the worst that can happen?"

PATIENT: "If he says no, I'll be stuck here for who knows how much longer."

STUDENT NURSE: "We can prepare for that then. I think we can find out how much longer specifically and go from there. I'll also check to see when the test is scheduled. I'll be glad to call the doctor and see what he says. Or if you want to call, I'll back you up."

PATIENT: "I sure would appreciate it if you'd call for me."

In this scenario, the nurse didn't get caught up in the negativism and kept a positive attitude by asking "what if" or "why not." Suggest whatever options are available in the situation using "what if" and "why not" phrases with people who are negative.

Another technique used to explain gently the nurse's different perception was the "to you, to me" approach. With this approach, you show that you are listening and then present your differing perception of the situation. You validate the viewpoint of the patient by restating it with a "to you" statement; then you add your own perception using the phrase "and to me."

The last technique used in this scenario is asking, "What is the worst that can happen?" Once people tell you the worst that can happen, you can help them prepare for whatever that might be.

In addition, as you talk with patients, try to avoid using the word "but." Use the word "and" instead. When you use "but," it erases whatever you said before it. Consider your interaction with a patient who's learning to give her own insulin. You say, "You've done a terrific job

COMMUNICATION

Competence Scale

DIRECTIONS: The questionnaire at right lists 20 personality characteristics. Please indicate the degree to which you believe each of these characteristics applies to YOU, as you normally communicate with others, by marking whether you...

(5) strongly agree that it applies,

(4) agree that it applies,

(3) are undecided,

(2) disagree that it applies, or

(1) strongly disagree that it applies.

There are no right or wrong answers.
Work quickly; record your first impression.

_____ 1. helpful
_____ 2. defends own beliefs
_____ 3. independent
_____ 4. responsive to others
_____ 5. forceful
_____ 6. has strong personality
_____ 7. sympathetic
_____ 8. compassionate
_____ 9. assertive
_____ 10. sensitive to the needs of others
_____ 11. dominant
_____ 12. sincere
_____ 13. gentle
_____ 14. willing to take a stand
_____ 15. warm
_____ 16. tender
_____ 17. friendly
_____ 18. acts as a leader
_____ 19. aggressive
_____ 20. competitive

SCORING DIRECTIONS

* **Items 2, 3, 5, 6, 9, 11, 14, 18, 19, and 20 measure assertiveness.** Add the scores on these items to get your assertiveness score. **Items 1, 4, 7, 8, 10, 12, 13, 15, 16, and 17 measure responsiveness.** Add the scores on these items to get your responsiveness score.

SCORING DIRECTIONS

1. Plot your assertiveness score on the vertical line of the graph on page 127.

2. Plot your responsiveness score on the horizontal line of the graph on page 127.

3. Draw a line between the assertiveness and responsiveness points on the graph on page 127.

4. Whichever quadrant the line crosses indicates your typical communication pattern in most situations.

If you are not in quadrant 1, do not despair. You can learn to become more assertive and more responsive. It takes much practice.

A communication competence scale. (Reprinted by permission of Waveland Press, Inc. from McCroskey, JC and Richmond, VP: Fundamentals of Human Communication. Waveland Press, Prospect Heights, Illinois, 1996. All rights reserved. Redrawn.)

with drawing up medicine, but you now need to work on giving the injection to yourself." What you've done is negate the positive comment you made about how well the patient drew up the medicine. If you substitute "and" for "but," you've made a much more positive statement about what needs to be done next. The statement, "You've done a terrific job with drawing up medicine, and you now need to work on giving the injection to yourself," sounds so much better. Just one word made a big difference.[4]

SUMMARY

It is important to recognize that therapeutic communication involves assertiveness and responsiveness, and that the situation dictates the appropriate amounts of each to be used.

It is very challenging for student nurses to learn to be assertive and responsive with patients. There are basic therapeutic communication strategies that must be mastered to do so.

First, describe the behavior, what the person is doing that is a problem. Always focus on what the person is doing behaviorally, not who they are. Actively listen to the contents of the message. Describe what you are thinking and feeling with "I" statements such as "I feel, I want, I believe, It seems to me that," and so on. Make empathic statements to get at the emotions in the situation, such as "I realize that you are very concerned about . . ."

Summarize what you believe to be the real issues related to the patient's behaviors, and validate them with the patient. Develop a plan to solve the problem that was at the root of the behaviors. If you don't have a plan that might work, then you need to say, "I need to think about this for a few minutes" or "I need to consult with your physician (or whomever) and see what we can come up with to help in this situation." Make sure that the patient is agreeable with the plan to solve the problem.

In working with aggressive people who may be hostile and sarcastic, be careful not to become defensive. Don't react. Speak calmly and slowly, and get the person to sit down and talk about the problem. People with aggressive tendencies need to be in control of what is going on. When they're acting aggressively, they feel out of control. Present clear ideas as options, and the person will readily decide which plan of action is best.

With passive people who are too agreeable, make it easy for them to say no. Check to make sure that what you're asking the person to do is realistic, and check with him regularly to make sure he's keeping up with the plan that you both agreed on. Work with him to set realistic deadlines and prevent procrastination. Don't put a lot of pressure on him to make decisions; instead, give him time to think once you've presented the options.

For patients who have responsive patterns of communication, be sure to take a personal interest in their lives. For a task-oriented person, this approach may be considered an invasion of privacy and a waste of their time. Try to get right to the point with task-oriented people.

With all patients, you must listen with empathy to the patient's perception of the problem. Then explain your perceptions of the problem. Finally, acknowledge the problem and discuss differences and similarities between your perceptions and the patient's. Summarize and validate all impressions with the patient. Make recommendations, and ask for the patient's agreement. Make sure that it's easy for the patient to say no because most patients tend to assume agreeable, passive, placating roles with healthcare providers. They also tend to procrastinate and not follow through with what they say they'll do.

Nonadherence to the advice of a healthcare provider is commonplace. Adherence to recommendations has been shown to correlate with the patient's ability to participate in developing plans of care, not just being told, "This is what you need to do."[10] The application of principles of therapeutic communication during patient education is covered in Chapter 9.

COMMUNICATION EXERCISES

1 Use the figure on page 140 as a self-assessment test to determine how assertive and responsive you are to others. Once you have completed the exercise, add up your points and fill in the grid on page 127.

2 Think about your last encounter with a person whose behavior upset you. The person does not have to be a patient. Describe the person's behavior and your behavior. What could you have done differently in the situation?

3 Write three comments about the behaviors of the person who upset you that you could give without making the person feel attacked.

4 In what situations do you get angry? How do you control your anger? Respond in terms of aggression and passivity or assertiveness and responsiveness.

5 What therapeutic communication strategies can you use to avoid a verbal battle with an aggressive person?

6 What therapeutic communication strategies can you use to get a passive person to tell you if she can't do something that you've asked of her?

References

1. Satir, V: The New Peoplemaking. Science and Behavior Books: Mountain View, California, 1988.
2. Lachman, VD: Taming your anger. Nursing 98 *28:*61, 1998.
3. Bem, SL: The measurement of psychological androgyny. Journal of Consulting and Clinical Psychology *42:*155, 1974.
4. Dymer, C: How to Handle Difficult People. National Press Publications, Overland Park, Kansas, 1992.
5. Wheeless, VE, and Dierks-Stewart, K: The psychometric properties of the Bem sex-role inventory: Questions concerning reliability and validity. Communication Quarterly *29:*173, 1981.
6. Selye, H: The Stress of Life. Mcgraw-Hill, New York, 1976.
7. Herman, SJ: Becoming Assertive: A Guide for Nurses. D. Van Nostrand, New York, 1978.
8. Milstead, JA: Basic tools for the orthopaedic staff nurse. Part 1: Assertiveness. Orthopaedic Nursing *15:*23, 1996.
9. Szasz, TS, and Hollender, HM: A contribution to the philosophy of medicine: The basic models of the doctor-patient relationship. Am Soc Rev *97:*585, 1956.
10. Allshouse, KD: Treating patients as individuals. In Gerteis, M (ed): Through the Patient's Eyes: Understanding and Promoting Patient-Centered Care. Jossey-Bass, San Francisco, 1993.
11. McCroskey, JC, and Richmond, VP: Fundamentals of Human Communication. Waveland Press, Prospect Heights, Illinois, 1996.
12. Lazarus, AA: Assertion behavior: A brief note. Behavioral Therapy *4:*697, 1973.

Encouraging Emotional Release Using Touch: Cultural Implications

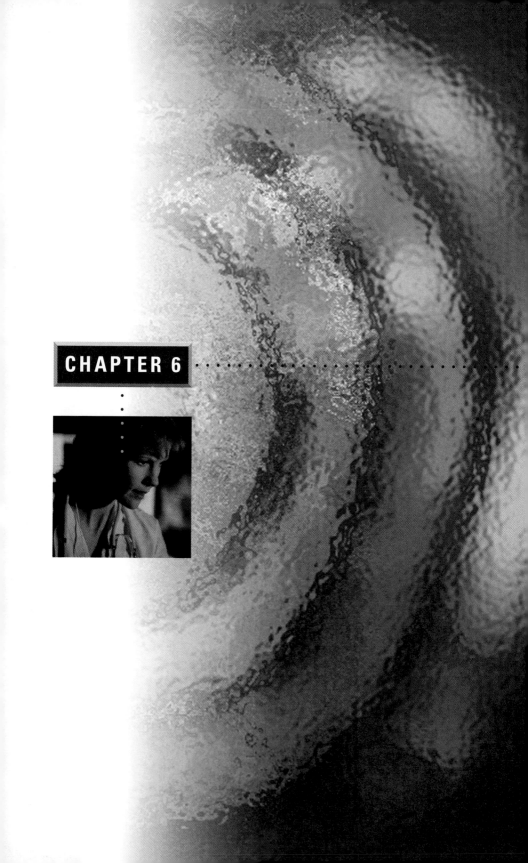

CHAPTER 6

Encouraging Emotional Release Using Touch: Cultural Implications

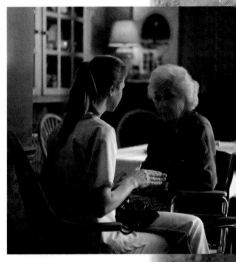

Chapter Objectives

AFTER READING THIS CHAPTER,
YOU WILL BE ABLE TO:

1. Identify why touch is a basic form of human communication.
2. Describe the basic human need for touch throughout life.
3. Identify the three basic forms of touch used by nurses.
4. Describe the cultural implications of touch.
5. Define proxemics and the four zones of personal space.
6. Identify appropriate nursing behaviors in each zone of personal space.
7. Distinguish between situations when touch is and is not acceptable.
8. Describe the physiological and psychological benefits of touch.

THE PRIMARY PURPOSE OF THIS CHAPTER IS TO HELP YOU DEVELOP AN understanding of touch and how to use it effectively in nursing practice. Touch is an important communication skill and a critical part of administering nursing care. Some nurses find it difficult to rationalize spending time holding a patient's hand or massaging a patient's back when staff is short and so many technological tasks need to be done. These are task-oriented, technological nurses; most have put caring touches in a closet. Other nurses believe all forms of touch are indispensable nursing interventions.[1]

Nursing has always been a very "high-touch" profession. Nurses must learn how and when to touch, as well as when not to touch. Touch is the most basic form of human nonverbal communication. Through touch, humans communicate such emotions as love, anger, and fear. Depending on our age and cultural upbringing, we may demonstrate our love by a hug or kiss. In anger, we may become aggressive, jabbing a finger in someone's chest or slapping the person. In fear, we may cling to each other. In childhood, we see the raw forms of emotional expression through touch. As adults, we learn to control the way we touch to express our emotions through socialization. We attempt to act in culturally acceptable ways to express our feelings through touch.

Nurses use three basic forms of touch, sometimes touching patients in very intimate ways.[1-3] You'll use emotionally supportive, caring touches to help a patient express herself, to comfort a patient during emotional distress, to show a patient that he is valued and respected, and to gain a patient's cooperation. You'll use procedural task touches to perform technical care. For example, recent nursing research indicates that you can significantly decrease the pain of an injection by pressing the site with your thumb, hard enough to feel resistance, and maintaining the pressure for 10 seconds.[4] You'll also use protective touches to keep patients from harming themselves, others, or you.

Touching Takes Practice

Most nursing students are anxious about touching patients. They're awkward and embarrassed about viewing and touching the typically unexposed "private parts" of human anatomy and touching patients in intimate areas. For example, in fundamentals courses, students typically are hesitant and anxious about performing basic procedures, such as a bed bath. They're awkward when picking up a patient's arm to put on a blood pressure cuff. When learning health assessment, a male student may wonder in embarrassment what he's supposed to do with a woman's breast while he tries to find her apical pulse. In addition, many students lack knowledge and self-confidence in how to touch patients who are emotionally distressed, in pain, anxious, or agitated.

Anxiety and awkward behaviors are typical, natural reactions whenever anyone does something new. As you gain practice in touching patients, you'll become much more comfortable doing so, even when you need to touch patients intimately. You also will develop your own professional therapeutic touching style. It comes partly from what you already know about touching.

Touch is a special form of nonverbal communication that we have all experienced. As with any communication technique, some of us are better at using and interpreting touches than others. The way you have learned to touch other humans is the result of your life experiences and cultural influences. Research has also shown that children of "high-touch" families are touchers as adults.[5,6] In conducting informal classroom surveys, I have found students of Italian, Jewish, Spanish, and South American ethnic backgrounds to report touching more frequently than students of German and British ancestry. To research public displays of touch, Sidney Jourard counted the number of touches per hour among couples sitting in cafes in various countries. He found 180 touches per hour in Puerto Rico, 110 touches per hour in Paris, two touches per hour in Gainesville, Florida, and no touches per hour in London.[7] These findings illustrate the influence of culture on touch.

In general, North Americans are very careful about whom they touch. Reasons for this reticence include the fear that a touch may be misinterpreted as having sexual overtones or perceived as controlling.[8] People also worry about accusations of sexual harassment and abuse in schools and workplaces. A slogan of the National Education Association, whose membership includes millions of teachers, sums up the sad situation in North America today: "Teach, don't touch." In contrast, we've all observed politicians spending a lot of time shaking hands and hugging in crowds of people. Does reaching out and touching people help get these politicians elected? They seem to think so. In addition, research has indicated that waitresses who touched customers on the shoulder or hand as they returned change received bigger tips than those who didn't.[9]

Touch: A Basic Human Need

Touch is a basic human need, as necessary for survival as food, clothing, and shelter. It is the first sense to develop in humans and is with us until death. In 1248, German emperor Frederick II was curious to see what language children would speak if no one talked to them or cuddled them. He conducted his "research" by taking newborns from their parents and having "nurses" feed them without talking to them or cuddling them. The babies all died before speaking because of the lack of touch.[9]

In the 1940s, Spitz reviewed orphanage records and found that orphans were more likely to die in the first years of life than other children were.[10] These findings led to the closing of many orphanages; they were replaced by foster homes, where children lived until they could be placed for adoption. Unfortunately, this finding that children fail to thrive without tactile and verbal stimulation was again confirmed in the 1990s in Romania, when thousands of infants, virtually abandoned in their orphanage cribs for 2 years, were severely impaired.[9]

A series of classic scientific experiments by Harlow further documents the importance of touch in primates.[11] He isolated newborn monkeys from their mothers and found that, given a choice between food and a terry cloth figure resembling their mother, the infant monkeys chose the terry cloth "mother." This demonstrated the instinctive drive these animals had for contact. Reite demonstrated that young monkeys taken from their mothers searched frantically and made distress sounds. Then, in a day or two, they gave up, sat slouched with sad faces, and didn't play.[12] These studies imply that human and primate infants, not as developed at birth as other mammals, are especially in need of touch.

It is important to recognize your own cultural beliefs about the importance of touch. For example, say that you've fed and changed a 6-month-old baby and you lay her in her crib for a nap. You've done everything you can think of to prepare the baby for her nap, and she's not sick in any way. But the baby starts to cry when you lay her down. Would your mother and family tell you to hold and rock the baby, to let the baby cry to exercise her lungs, or to ignore the crying to avoid spoiling the child? At present, child authorities generally advise picking up a baby when it cries to meet the child's security needs and ultimately affect the child's self-concept. In other words, the child learns that she can trust others and that she is important, resulting in a positive self-concept.[8] Recent studies of massage in premature infants by Field have shown that a 15-minute massage three times daily led to hospital discharge 6 days early, at a savings of $10,000 per infant.[13,14] Other studies have shown that handling increases visual alertness in babies and also has soothing effects.[15,16]

Touch also supplies the security needed for exploration as a toddler. Children explore their environment and repeatedly run back to their mothers for reassurance when frightened. After consolation, they feel secure to return to their exploration. Touch provides infants with security necessary for normal psychological development and self-concept.[12,15] The happy and secure infant has had his need for touch met.

Doesn't it follow that, as people grow into adults, they still need touch? However, although the need for touch doesn't go away, it may be neglected and ignored by adults. Hollender conducted interviews of men and women to determine the adult desire to hold or be held.[17,18] Most people indicated a moderate desire to be held, with men nearly as high as women in their ratings of the desire to hold or to be held. He found that many adults reported an increased need for touch when they were depressed or anxious.

The Physiological Response of the Body to Touch

Touch can be used to decrease a patient's response to stress. Whenever a person feels apprehension and pain, the body launches a stress response, a sequence of biochemical events. The perception of stress by the cortex and hypothalamus of the brain activates the interactive autonomic nervous system, the psychoneuroendocrine system, and the musculoskeletal system.[19]

Touch focuses on affecting the musculoskeletal system. A well-known effect of stress is increased muscular tension and rigidity. Motor pathways of the autonomic nervous system stimulate the musculoskeletal system, along with stimulation by hormones from the psychoneuroendocrine system. Touch transmits messages to the brain to calm the stress response. Indeed, the skin contains millions of touch receptors—up to 3000 in just a fingertip—that send messages along the spinal cord to the brain. Once these messages arrive, the brain regulates the autonomic and psychoneuroendocrine systems. Endorphins , which are the body's natural way of suppressing pain, are produced. Also, production of cortisol and norepinephrine decreases. Cortisol suppresses immune functioning, and norepinephrine prepares us for the fight-or-flight response by increasing heart rate, blood pressure, and breathing.

A simple, caring touch to a shoulder or the feel of an arm around a waist can reduce the heart rate and lower blood pressure. That's why a mother's hugging a child with a skinned knee may actually make it better from a physiological standpoint. In addition, massage stimulates the vagus nerve, resulting in the release of glucose and insulin, hormones that promote food absorption.[9,20] That's why premature babies gain weight faster and leave the hospital sooner when they receive regular massage.[13,14] Following exercise, massage can also stimulate the flow of blood and lymph to and from muscles, thus releasing lactic acid buildup, removing toxins, and alleviating pain and congestion in muscles.[21] The bottom line is that touch, when it is administered effectively, stimulates a relaxation response in the body.

Nurses Use Touch

Nurses have social permission to touch people. The social permission cuts across all cultures. In other words, patients expect nurses to touch them. Social permission means that people will allow and actually expect nurses to touch them during procedures. They also allow and expect nurses to provide comforting touches. Touching is part of the nurse's job description. The beginning nursing student typically wonders if patients will trust her and allow her to touch them when performing procedures and offering comfort. Prepare for a pleasant surprise: Most people like to be touched. Most patients willingly accept and like nurses and nursing students very much, and welcome touches from them.

The primary factor that determines how a patient will respond to touch is the intention of the touch. Jones suggests that touch needs to be related to the context of the situation.[5,8] The meaning of the touch relates to the situation, the timing, and the manner in which the touch is delivered. You will need to evaluate each situation carefully for touch opportunities and then deliver appropriate touches depending on what occurs in the clinical situation. Thus, a hand on a patient's shoulder can convey, "I want to comfort you," "I like you," or "I was just kidding."

You need to become familiar with the three basic forms of touch that have been identified in nursing: caring touch, task touch, and protective touch. You also need to know when it's appropriate to use and not to use touch.[1–3]

CARING TOUCH

Caring touch has an emotional intent and involves comforting touch and encouraging touch. Comforting touch includes holding a patient's hand, stroking his forehead, squeezing his shoulder, stroking his arm, and placing a hand on his chest. These types of touches are usually associated with dying, discomfort, or grief. Specifically, patients who are in pain, anxious, frightened, confused, or agitated often respond very positively to touch. They will openly express their appreciation and reciprocate the touch. For example, consider the family member who reported that his wife's favorite nurse spent a few minutes each day holding her hand and stroking her forehead when she was very ill during chemotherapy for breast cancer. He described her as the "best nurse" because of how much she cared about his wife as a person.

Encouraging touches include placing an arm around the shoulders, giving a hug or a pat on the back, and playful hitting and poking. Encouraging touch is more hopeful and future oriented, and is often used to celebrate clinical progress. These touches are used for supporting, reassuring, and raising the spirits of patients and families. For example, several hours after nursing a patient through a difficult labor, a labor and delivery nurse visits a patient and asks how she's doing and immediately gives her a hug. The hug conveys congratulations and also emotional support at that special time. Other clinical research applications for caring touch indicate that hand holding before anesthesia usually makes the procedure less frightening. In other operating room examples, a nurse may stand at the foot of the bed and lay a hand on the foot or ankle of the patient or may stand at the head of the bed and lay a hand on the patient's face to reduce the patient's anxiety.[22]

TASK TOUCH

Most touch in nursing is task touch involving physical assessment and procedural treatments that must be done. The objective is to be as gentle, soft, and careful with task touches as you can be. In other words, task touch should overlap with caring touch. Through slow, gentle, soft, and careful touch during assessments and procedures, you will communicate warmly that you value and respect patients, and you really do care about them. In contrast, hurried, rough, jarring touches communicate coldness and uncaring.

Gender differences in touch have been the focus of studies. Characteristically, men are less gentle when touching others than women are.[23] All students, male and female, must learn to touch gently and carefully. Hurried, rough, jarring touches convey a lack of respect for the patient, almost as if the patient were an inanimate object without feelings, as depicted in the cartoon on page 154.

The same husband who described his wife's "best nurse" as using caring touch also described her "worst nurse" as one that didn't care. This nurse would come in to the room and focus on doing the task at hand, such as changing an intravenous solution, while barely glancing at the patient. She hurried to finish and leave as quickly as possible. One day this nurse came to work with a bad cold. The husband became irate and went to the administrator, refusing to let the nurse in the room to ever care for his wife again. He realized that his wife's chemotherapy affected her blood counts and made her very susceptible to infection. He was right. And he felt even more strongly that the nurse didn't care about his wife.

PROTECTIVE TOUCH

Physically protective touches for patients involve the issue of control over the patient and the situation in which patient safety is a primary concern. It is best to combine protective touch with caring touch whenever possible. For example, patients sometimes need to be held down to keep them from harming themselves. Confused patients may be restrained and sedated to ensure that they won't pull on vital tubes or fall out of a bed or chair. It is often helpful to use caring touch with a patient who is being restrained. The patient's hand can be gently held down as someone else carefully applies the restraint.

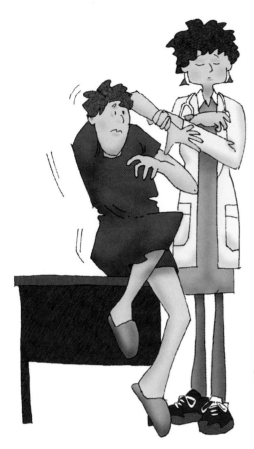

Hurried, rough, jarring touches convey a lack of respect for the patient, almost as if the patient were an inanimate object without feelings.

Take care, though, to minimize the danger of being hurt by a combative patient who may attempt to strike or harm you. Say, for example, that an elderly woman who had gallbladder surgery has a reaction to the anesthetic. She becomes disoriented, doesn't know where she is, and attempts to pull out her intravenous line and get out of bed. She is very strong, and it takes two male attendants to hold her down while you gently apply restraints. The next morning, when the anesthetic has worn off and she is fully alert, you can safely remove the restraints.

Inhibition of Nursing Touch

The lack of touch and the use of task touch without adding caring touches has been described as emotionally protective to the nurse. Nursing research suggests that nurses who are task oriented may be distancing themselves from pain and suffering as a means to protect themselves emotionally.[1,2] The nurse may be suffering from burnout, which creates a negative attitude about the work environment. He may be emotionally and physically exhausted, resulting in a negative self-concept. And he may feel a loss of concern for the patient and family.[24] The burned out nurse has little or no emotional energy to relate to patients. In general, the better the nurse feels physically and emotionally, the better his ability to relate to patients by touch or any other communication technique. Burnout and its prevention are discussed in Chapter 4.

Harsh or severe touches have also been related to the nurse's emotional protection as a means to release tension. Nurses who are unable to communicate effectively, either verbally or nonverbally, with confused and agitated patients become frustrated. Frustration leads to tensions that must be released. Nurses may have feelings of reaching the "end of the rope," and quickly move to sedate and restrain patients, using harsh touches that release their own emotional tension.[2]

In addition, research indicates that some patient characteristics decrease the amount of caring touches administered to them.[2] Some patients are much more difficult to establish therapeutic relationships with than others, depending on whether or not the nurse likes the patient. Realistically, you will not like every one of your patients. You will not be able to relate well to every patient. For example, patients with behavioral problems—such as those who are demanding, verbally abusive, and uncooperative—receive less caring touch and more protective touch. Those with contagious diseases, such as acquired immunodeficiency syndrome (AIDS) or tuberculosis, receive fewer touches because of the nurse's fear of acquiring the disease. Also, patients perceived as responsible for their own conditions, such as alcoholics or drug addicts who repeatedly overdose, typically receive less touch.[2] It's ironic that these patients receive less touch because they are the ones most in need of caring touch and other forms of emotional support. These are the stigmatized outcasts of society. Usually, they have the worst self-concepts, and they think that nobody likes them and nobody wants to associate with them. Sometimes, appropriate touch can help to improve the self-concept for these patients because touch demonstrates acceptance and support.

Getting Started with Touch

The best way to find out if a patient is receptive to touch is to try it. Begin with a handshake when you first meet your patient. Watch the patient's reaction carefully. Look for grimacing or body tensing. Note whether the patient pulls away, lets her hand linger, or even clings to your hand.

If you care for that patient on a second day, again offer a handshake to greet her formally and to show warmth and respect. One student reported that an elderly woman patient was so starved for touch that the patient literally climbed up her arm and pulled her down into the bed to give her a hug!

SHAKING HANDS

Handshaking has become a means of communicating how we feel about each other. In North America, we estimate the warmth and sincerity of a person by how they shake hands. We have all experienced the variations of handshakes, including differences in pressure, duration, and awkwardness. Chances are that you already understand the rules of the customary handshake in Western civilizations. Emily Post says that the handshake should be firm, with slightly more firmness for a close friend.[25] A hearty, firm grip is supposed to indicate that you are sincere and pleased to meet someone. Men usually have a stronger handshake grip than women.[23]

Look the person in the eyes and smile as you shake their hand. Expressions that are used with the handshake include, "Glad to meet you" or "How are you today?" Some people return this "textbook" shake by shaking hands and at the same time grasping the elbow or forearm of the other person's arm. A few grasp the extended hand with both hands and shake. Both variations indicate extra affection and friendliness.[9]

In America, a limp handshake is considered a cool reception and unfriendly, whereas a viselike, crushing handshake carries the intent to intimidate.[8] The handshake is a clue to the person's attitude about himself and others.

In general, handshakes are required as you meet someone for the first time, whether you introduce yourself or are introduced by someone else. In the past, men alone shook hands, not women. Today women are expected to shake hands when they are introduced to each other or to men.

When departing, handshakes can also be done, but these shakes do not have to be as formal as when you first met your patient. More typically, after working with a patient intimately for a day, you can just take his hand in yours and squeeze it, and tell him it was very nice being with him today and you look forward to seeing him again. If you will not see the patient again, then you need to wish the person well and good luck, and tell him you hope everything works out for him.

Suppose you've just met your patient for the day, shaken hands, and noted that the patient held on to your hand for a few seconds longer than you would have otherwise expected. She smiled at you as you shook her hand. Both the lingering hand and the smile lets you know she responded to your touch positively.

Next, you do a brief physical assessment to be sure she is progressing physically as expected, and then discuss plans for how to proceed with the tasks that need to be done that day. You begin by pulling back the sheets and lift her gown. The patient frowns, clings to her covers and says, "What are you going to do to me?" What went wrong?

ENTERING PERSONAL SPACE

You violated rules for entering personal space by pulling back her covers without asking permission and without using anticipatory guidance. You need to be very aware of personal space, and the rules that apply when moving about within the personal space of each individual. We all dearly protect our personal space. This space is an invisible bubble that surrounds each of us. Proxemics involves the study of personal space, and the meaning of proximity or closeness of one person to another as the distance between the two people increases or decreases. The space has four zones: intimate, personal, social, and public.[26]

The Intimate Zone

The intimate zone of personal space is from the skin surface to about 16 inches away. This is the zone that was violated in the earlier example. People guard this zone the most. This zone is reserved for close friends and relatives, to those with whom there is emotional closeness. Nurses and other healthcare providers must ask permission to enter the intimate zone.

Make sure you tell a person what you're going to do *before* you attempt to do anything inside the intimate zone. Explain sensations that the patient can expect to feel as you touch him so he won't think that he's experiencing anything out of the ordinary. Explaining the steps and sensations in a procedure as you go along is called anticipatory guidance.

Warm your hands and your stethoscope before touching the patient. Nothing makes someone tense up and withdraw faster than cold hands. Use slow, deliberate, gentle, and purposeful touches as you do your assessment or any procedure, watching the patient's nonverbal responses. Always ask permission and let the patient know what you'll be doing before you touch, even for the simplest procedure, such as a blood pressure.

The Personal Zone

A bit farther out, from 1.5 to 4 feet, is the personal zone. This is generally the most used zone. When not in a healthcare setting, it is used for socializing. People typically stand this far from others at parties and friendly gatherings. In nursing, this is the zone in which to conduct a personal history as well as to discuss plans for how to proceed with the activities that must be done on any given day. Sit on the same level with the patient and discuss the plan and options quietly. If one person sits and the other stands, the person standing has a position of dominance, and also gives the impression of not having much time to sit and discuss the plan of care. If you want to find out if the patient is having any problems or feeling any discomfort, you need to move to within 4 feet and get on the same level as the patient.

That sounds simple enough, but here is an example of what happens in reality. Your clinical instructor routinely monitors the care that you give to the patient each day on the clinical unit. The clinical instructor walks over to your patient, you introduce her, and she shakes the patient's hand. The instructor looks at your charting documentation to date and notices that you wrote that the patient had "No reports of discomfort." The instructor next asks the patient, "How are things going?" followed by, "Is anything bothering you? Are you comfortable?"

The patient responds with, "My back is aching this morning, and I didn't sleep good last night."

The instructor now looks at you for an explanation of why you didn't pick up on this. You look at your instructor in amazement and say, "I just asked him, and he said he was feeling fine."

You may have been too far away, outside the personal zone, when you asked how he was doing. This rather embarrassing and awkward situation has happened many times to many students. The lesson to be learned here is to be sure to get within 4 feet of the patient when asking personal questions. Beginning students need to get accustomed to being in this personal zone with a person who would otherwise be a stranger. Typically, you wouldn't stand so close to a stranger.

There is, however, a different set of expectations about how you should act in the role of nurse. One of those expectations is that you are within personal distance most of the time, especially if you want to develop effective interpersonal relationships and encourage patients to respond to you as you would like them to. Combine effective use of the personal zone with active listening, and you're well on your way to developing an effective helping relationship with a patient.

The Social Zone

From 4 to 12 feet away from a person is the social zone. This is an impersonal zone, and it's the space used for strangers and for people we do not know. This zone is often misused in nursing. Most of what we do in nursing requires the use of the personal zone because what we discuss is private.

When you stand in the social zone to discuss personal matters, you give the impression of being impersonal and not caring. For example, imagine a nurse who stands in the doorway of a semiprivate room and announces to Mrs. Jones in Bed A that it's time for her enema. Mrs. Jones would much rather have kept her bowel status personal, and would be embarrassed by the announcement and probably upset with the nurse for being insensitive. The nurse should have used the personal zone.

The Public Zone

Distances that exceed 12 feet from a person are in the public zone. A person giving a speech would stand at least 12 feet from the audience. You might use the public zone during patient educational activities that involve giving a lecture to a group of patients and their families.

The above-mentioned generalizations about personal space are based on research involving European North Americans. The distances in the four zones are averages that have been computed based on observations of North Americans. Keep in mind that different cultures draw different lines around personal space. So, depending on your ethnic background, you or your patient may need more or less personal space.

For example, those of us who are descendants of Hispanics, Middle Easterners, and Southern Europeans (Italians, French, Spanish, and so on) stand much closer and feel comfortable when people stand close to us. Those of us whose ancestors were from Asia and Northern Europe (Germany, England, Ireland, and so on) may not feel as comfortable having someone stand close to us, and are used to having more space.

You've probably experienced having someone who was not a close personal friend stand so close that it made you feel uncomfortable. Perhaps you backed away from the person and he followed you and got "in your face" again. When a member of a close-contact cultural background moves in next to you, it's important to stand your ground in as relaxed a way as possible, and learn to calm yourself. In contrast, if someone is backing away and seems to be trying to keep you at arm's length, don't follow. Let the person have the space he needs. Although you need to keep the intimate, personal, social, and public zones ingrained in your mind and the behaviors expected within the zones, temper that knowledge with the fact that you must allow the patient and family to select the distance that is comfortable to them when they are talking to you.

GIVING PAINFUL TOUCHES

One rule that transcends all cultures is to never inflict pain on another through touch, even accidentally.[8] For example, if your sister accidentally steps on your foot, you most likely immediately react with something like, "Ouch, be careful, you just smashed my foot!" Your sister would probably apologize immediately.

As you know, however, some nursing procedures are uncomfortable and some hurt. Many students feel bad about purposefully performing procedures that hurt. For example, dressing changes, suture removal, injections, catheterizations, and so on can be uncomfortable. First, you must learn the correct way to perform each procedure so that it produces the least amount of pain. And you must use pain medication appropriately before painful procedures. Talk gently and use anticipatory guidance as you do a procedure.

Avoid giving patients the impression that they are objects to be worked on. If a procedure requires your full attention, a second person should be available strictly for emotional support and anticipatory guidance of the patient. For example, it may take two people to peform a catheterization, one to support the patient and the other to do the procedure. Apologize during and after the procedure, "I know that this hurts, but I will be done in a minute. Thank you for holding so still." Afterward, "I'm sorry I hurt you. You were very patient and cooperative."

HUGGING

Nurses can learn to give compassionate and supportive hugs that are thoughtful and respectful. Hugs can be therapeutic when the intention of the hug is to show that you care and want to comfort a patient or family member of the patient.[25] Hugging a child before the induction of anesthesia may make it less frightening, for example. Hugs can be comforting for adults as well.

As you read this, you might be thinking, "What about the sexual overtones of a hug?" Hugs that nurses dispense are compassionate, not passionate. Patients recognize the difference. However, be certain that you have permission before hugging. A hug is within the intimate zone and, therefore, requires permission. Sometimes the permission may be nonverbal and you respond spontaneously. Or you could ask, "Can I give you a hug?"

Also, recognize that there are many types of hugs for different purposes. You'll develop your own hugging style and a sense for when a hug is needed and acceptable. Keating, in her book on hug therapy, described 10 types of hugs.[27] Three hugs that I have found to be especially useful in nursing situations include the A-frame hug, the side-to-side hug, and the bear hug, as shown in the cartoon on page 162.

A-Frame Hug

The A-frame hug involves wrapping two arms around the shoulders of the patient and leaning in toward the patient until your shoulders and cheeks touch. This hug is brief, and nothing below the shoulders makes contact. Patients may also wrap their arms around your shoulders. If you have not had much experience hugging, this is a comfortable and nonthreatening hug to try first.

This hug is classic and formal, and can also be used with new acquaintances or professional colleagues. It is often used in some cultures as a hello or goodbye hug, and may be combined with a kiss on the cheek. So, for example, say that a patient you've worked with for a week is ready for discharge to home. As you say goodbye, this is a good hug to use. This hug may be accompanied by back patting.

Side-to-Side Hug

The side-to-side hug is a one armed squeeze around the shoulder or the waist of another. It is a more playful hug. Suppose you are walking with a patient, supporting her around the shoulders or waist. As you help her back into bed, you might give her a squeeze and tell her what a good job she did walking and that she's making good progress. If the patient is crying or frightened, you may gently put an arm around her shoulders or waist to offer emotional support.

Bear Hug

Bear hugs are those in which bodies touch in a powerful, strong squeeze that can last for 5 to 10 seconds and give a warm, supportive, secure feeling. Take care to make the hug firm and not breathless, remembering always to be considerate of your partner.

Parents share these hugs with children, giving a "You are terrific" message. Friends might give these hugs as a way to share joy or sorrow. For example, this hug may be a way of sharing the joy with a friend on a happy occasion such as marriage or when two people have not seen each other in a long time. It may also be a way of sharing sorrow, as during the funeral of a loved one.

Bear hugs can be used therapeutically to raise self-esteem. In fact, they're used therapeutically during group meetings of Alcoholics

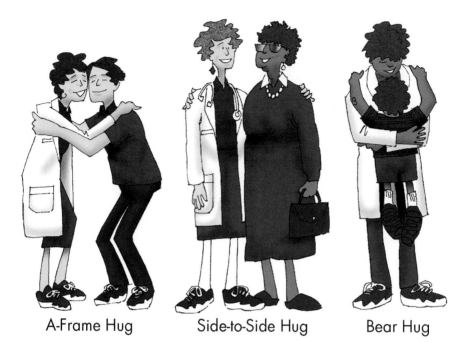

| A-Frame Hug | Side-to-Side Hug | Bear Hug |

Types of hugs. "Hugging is healthy. It helps the body's immunity system, keeps you healthier, eases depression, reduces stress, induces sleep, invigorates, rejuvenates, and causes no unpleasant side effects. It's nothing less than a miracle drug. Hugging is also all natural. It's organic, naturally sweet, pesticide-free, preservative-free, and 100% wholesome with no artificial ingredients.

*In fact, hugging is practically perfect. There are no moving parts, no batteries to wear out, and no periodic checkups. It requires little energy and yields high energy. It's inflation-proof and nonfattening. It demands no monthly payments and no insurance requirements. And it's theft-proof, nontaxable, nonpolluting, and, of course, fully returnable." (*Author unknown*)*

Anonymous. People with alcoholism often have very low self-esteem. At the beginning of meetings, group members welcome each other and newcomers to the group with group bear hugs to show support and caring.

RULES FOR WHEN AND HOW NOT TO TOUCH

A patient with a history of abuse, either physical or sexual, may prefer little or no touch beyond what is needed to carry out tasks. Psychiatric patients may require special care with touch. Patients will keep their distance and pull away to avoid a touch. If you wake up a schizophrenic patient by touching him, shaking his arm for example, he may react violently. If you call out his name first, then ask permission to touch him, the response will be much calmer.[1]

Nurses must become very sensitive to patients who withdraw from touch. If a patient withdraws as you touch him and you realize that you made a touch mistake, offer a brief apology, such as, "I'm sorry, I didn't mean to startle you." Your apology shows that you care and that you are aware of what happened.

Avoid touches that are sexually stimulating in nature. For instance, touches that are overly long for the intended purpose have been associated with sexual interest.[1,7] Sometimes, even caring touch may cause sexual arousal in a patient. If this happens, limit your touches to task touches, keeping them gentle and unhurried. This usually prevents further problems. If the problem persists, you may need to speak with the patient about it.[1]

Many students are concerned that patients may misinterpret their touches, even during a procedure. For example, young female students just learning to do bed baths commonly express concern about male patients becoming sexually stimulated during cleaning of the genitals. Likewise, male students express the same concerns as they learn to bathe females. My advice is to avoid long, lingering touches anywhere, especially in private areas. In addition, take comfort in the fact that the vast majority of patients unable to perform their own perineal care are too sick to become aroused. As you clean, focus on the idea that perineal care is essential to prevent urinary tract infections.

Massage: A Classic Touch Technique

Massage has been promoted as providing benefits to mind, body, and spirit. Massage techniques date back to ancient times, when Roman and Greek physicians used it to alleviate pain and promote healing, as well as to relax and tone muscles. At present, massage is very popular as a means to reduce stress and help with relaxation. Millions of Americans visit massage therapists yearly, and parents are learning how to give massages to their babies. Massages are even being offered in workplaces, including the U.S. Department of Justice. The medical research on massage is mounting, indicating that it has positive effects in many conditions, such as lowering anxiety in depressed adolescents, reducing agitation in Alzheimer's patients, easing stiffness and pain in arthritis sufferers, helping people with asthma breathe easier, and boosting immune functioning in AIDS patients.[9]

Nurses have traditionally given back massages as part of the morning bath procedure to stimulate circulation and reduce backaches in patients confined to bed. Back massages are also helpful in inducing relaxation when performed as part of the evening prepara-

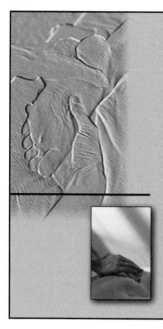

ACUPUNCTURE

Chinese practice of puncturing the body with needles at specific points in the skin to relieve discomfort and cure disease. [21]

ACUPRESSURE (SHIATSU)

Eastern practice involving a massage with the fingers applied to the specific areas of the skin used in acupuncture. [21]

REFLEXOLOGY

Egyptian practice of massaging the hands or feet based on the belief that pressure applied to specific points on these extremities benefits other parts of the body. [21]

THERAPEUTIC TOUCH

Practice in which, after the patient attains a meditative state, the hands of the therapeutic touch therapist are kept 2 to 6 inches from the body, where the energy fields of the touch therapist and the patient interact. The therapeutic touch therapist assesses for areas of discomfort, then directs healing energy toward the area of imbalance. [28]

Advanced touch therapies.

tion for sleep procedure. As described in many fundamental nursing texts, nurses learn to use a combination of techniques, including stroking, friction, pressure, and kneading for back messages. Many patients have opened up and talked about what is worrying them during or after a back massage. Although back rubs are not for everyone, many patients appreciate them and feel more secure following massages, believing that the nurse can be trusted and is interested in them.

A word of caution, however: If you aren't focused on what you are doing, if you are distracted, if you are just going through the motions, if you use rough and jarring and hurried movements, don't bother even attempting the massage. This massage will increase stress. In addition, remember that not everyone likes to be massaged. Always ask if the patient would like a back rub first, as you should always do when entering the intimate zone.

You may be interested in integrating many other forms of touch therapies into your practice. Examples of touch therapies include acupuncture, acupressure, reflexology, and therapeutic touch. These therapies are not usually included in basic nursing education programs. Nurses require special certification courses before trying these therapies on patients. These therapies are briefly defined above.

The Touch Avoidance Scale

DIRECTIONS:

This instrument is composed of 18 statements concerning feelings about touching other people and being touched. Please indicate the degree to which each statement applies to you by circling whether you:

(1) Strongly Disagree,

(2) Disagree,

(3) Are Undecided,

(4) Agree, or

(5) Strongly Agree with each statement.

While some of these statements may seem repetitious, take your time and try to be as honest as possible.

RATING

	Strongly Disagree	Disagree	Undecided	Agree	Strongly Agree

1. A hug from a same-sex friend is a true sign of friendship.	1	2	3	4	5
2. Opposite-sex friends enjoy it when I touch them.	1	2	3	4	5
3. I often put my arm around friends of the same sex.	1	2	3	4	5
4. When I see two people of the same sex hugging, it revolts me.	1	2	3	4	5
5. I like it when members of the opposite sex touch me.	1	2	3	4	5
6. People shouldn't be so uptight about touching persons of the same sex.	1	2	3	4	5
7. I think it is vulgar when members of the opposite sex touch me.	1	2	3	4	5
8. When a member of the opposite sex touches me, I find it unpleasant.	1	2	3	4	5
9. I wish I were free to show emotions by touching members of the same sex.	1	2	3	4	5
10. I'd enjoy giving a massage to an opposite-sex friend.	1	2	3	4	5
11. I enjoy kissing persons of the same sex.	1	2	3	4	5
12. I like to touch friends who are the same sex as I am.	1	2	3	4	5

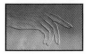

	Strongly Disagree	Disagree	Undecided	Agree	Strongly Agree
13. Touching a friend of the same sex does not make me uncomfortable.	1	2	3	4	5
14. I find it enjoyable when a close opposite-sex friend and I embrace.	1	2	3	4	5
15. I enjoy getting a backrub from a member of the opposite sex.	1	2	3	4	5
16. I dislike kissing relatives of the same sex.	1	2	3	4	5
17. Intimate touching with members of the opposite sex is pleasurable.	1	2	3	4	5
18. I find it difficult to be touched by a member of my own sex.	1	2	3	4	5

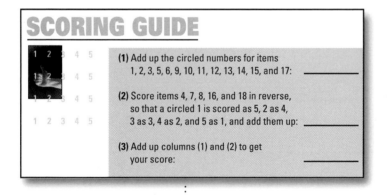

SCORING GUIDE

(1) Add up the circled numbers for items 1, 2, 3, 5, 6, 9, 10, 11, 12, 13, 14, 15, and 17: _____

(2) Score items 4, 7, 8, 16, and 18 in reverse, so that a circled 1 is scored as 5, 2 as 4, 3 as 3, 4 as 2, and 5 as 1, and add them up: _____

(3) Add up columns (1) and (2) to get your score: _____

70 AND ABOVE: *You have a strong motivation to touch. Only about 14% of people score this high.*

AROUND 60: *Your motivation to touch is average, but generally positive.*

54: *The score of 54 is the midpoint between positive and negative motivations regarding touch.*

50 OR BELOW: *You are below average in your motivation to touch. Only 14% of people score this low.*

Note: Item 15 from the original scale (Anderson & Leibowitz, 1978) has been altered from "when my date and I embrace" to "when a close opposite-sex friend and I embrace." Also, the scoring has been reversed from the original, so that a higher score indicates a more positive attitude toward touch.

The Touch Avoidance Scale. Adapted from scale originally developed by Anderson, PA and Leibowitz, K: The development and nature of the construct touch avoidance. Environmental Psychology and Nonverbal Behavior 3:89, 1978, published by Plenum Publishing Corporation, New York, New York. As appearing in Jones, SE: The Right Touch: Understanding and Using the Language of Physical Contact, Hampton Press Inc., Cresskill, New Jersey, 1994. Reprinted with permission.

SUMMARY

Nursing has a long history of employing touch to comfort and treat patients. The focus on technology has led to healthcare environments that are interpreted by patients as cold, uncaring, and dehumanizing. Many experienced nurses realize that touch can create a warm and caring atmosphere. Although staffing is minimal in most settings, it only takes a few minutes to hold a patient's hand or massage a back to demonstrate that you care about the patient and to promote relaxation.

Touch, a therapeutic communication skill that involves knowledge of how to touch and how not to touch, takes much practice. Touch involves personal sensitivity to patients and healthcare situations. If you combine effective use of touch with the other verbal communication techniques covered throughout the book, you are well on your way to helping patients control their response to stress and contributing to their health and healing. The patient's interpretation and perception of your use of touch and other verbal communication techniques directly affects whether or not the communication technique helps the patient to relax or creates more stress. As with any other communication technique, carefully monitor the patient's response to your touches and use these responses to guide further communications.

COMMUNICATION EXERCISES

1 Learning to touch should start with a personal assessment of your overall attitude toward touch. On page 165 is a questionnaire developed by Andersen and Leibowitz.[29] Although it is entitled the Touch Avoidance Scale, you can use it to find out how much you like to touch. The scale represents your attitude toward touch based on your past experiences.

2 Do this exercise in class as an introduction to the topic of touch. Go up to someone you do not know in class, shake hands, and introduce yourself. Follow this up with a group discussion of the various ways that students in class shook hands and what this means based on past experiences.

3 Give the partner you just met a hug. Experiment exchanging the A-frame, side-to-side, and bear hug with classmates. Follow the hugging with a group discussion of the type of hugs that were given in class and what this means based on your past experiences.

4 Give your partner a neck massage for 2 minutes, then switch around and receive a neck massage. Have a group discussion sharing different perceptions of how the massages felt and what it felt like to give a massage. Discuss differences in feelings depending on the level of intimacy of the touches.

References

1. Talton, CW: Touch—of all kinds—is therapeutic. RN *2:* 61, 1995.
2. Estabrooks, CA: Touch: A nursing strategy in the intensive care unit. Heart & Lung *18:*392,1989.
3. Adomat, R, and Killingworth, A: Care of the critically ill patient: The impact of stress on the use of touch in intensive therapy units. Journal of Advanced Nursing *19:*912,1994.
4. Barnhill BJ, et al: Using pressure to decrease the pain of intramuscular injections. Journal of Pain and Symptom Management *12:*52,1996.
5. Jones, SE, and Yarbrough, AE: A naturalistic study of the meanings of touch. Communication Monograph *52:*19,1985.
6. Gladney, K, and Barker, L: The effects of tactile history on attitudes toward and frequency of touching behavior. Sign Language Studies *24:*231,1979.
7. Jourard, SM: An exploratory study of body-accessibility. British Journal of Social & Clinical Psychology *5:*221,1966.
8. Jones, SE: The Right Touch: Understanding and Using the Language of Physical Contact. Hampton Press Inc., Cresskill, New Jersey, 1994.
9. Colt, GH, Schatz, H, and Hollister, A: The magic of touch. Life *8:*54–61,1997.
10. Spitz, RA: Anaclitic depression. Psycholytic Study of the Child *2:*313,1946.
11. Harlow, HF: The nature of love. American Psychologist *131:*673, 1958.
12. Reite, ML: Touch, attachment, and health: Is there a relationship? In Brown, CC (ed): The Many Facets of Touch. Johnson & Johnson Baby Products Company, 1984, p. 58.
13. Field, T, et al: Tactile/kinesthetic stimulation effects on preterm neonates. Pediatrics *77:*654,1986.
14. Field, T: Alleviating stress in newborn infants in the intensive care unit. Stimulation and the Preterm Infant *17:*1, 1990.
15. White, BL, and Castle, PW: Visual exploratory behavior following postnatal handling of human infants. Perceptual and Motor Skills *18:*497,1964.
16. Harrison, L, et al: Effects of gentle human touch on preterm infants: Pilot study results. Neonatal Network *15:*35,1996.
17. Hollender, MH: The need or wish to be held. Archives of General Psychiatry *22:*445,1970.

18. Hollender, MH: Wish to be held and wish to hold in men and women. Archives of General Psychiatry 33:49, 1976.
19. Wells-Federman, CL, et al: The mind-body connection: The psychophysiology of many traditional nursing interventions. Clinical Nurse Specialist 9:59, 1995.
20. Montagu, A: The Human Significance of the Skin, ed 3. Harper & Row, New York, 1986.
21. Kahn, S, and Saulo, M: Healing Yourself: A Nurse's Guide to Self-Care and Renewal. Delmar, Albany, New York, 1994.
22. Tovar, MK: Touch: The beneficial effects for the surgical patient. AORN J 49:1356, 1989.
23. Glass, L: He Says, She Says: Closing the Communication Gap Between the Sexes. Berkeley, New York, 1993.
24. Freudenberger, HJ: Staff burnout. Journal of Social Issues 30:159, 1974.
25. Post, E: Etiquette: The Blue Book of Social Usage. Funk & Wagnall, New York, 1940.
26. Hall, ET: The Hidden Dimension. Anchor Books/Doubleday, Garden City, NY, 1966.
27. Keating, K: The Hug Therapy Book. Hazelden, Center City, Minnesota, 1983.
28. Krieger, D: The Therapeutic Touch: How To Use Your Hands To Help or Heal. Prentice-Hall, Englewood Cliffs, NJ, 1979.
29. Anderson, PA and Leibowitz, K: The development and nature of the construct touch avoidance. Environmental Psychology and Nonverbal Behavior 3:89, 1978.

Encouraging Emotional Release Using Humor

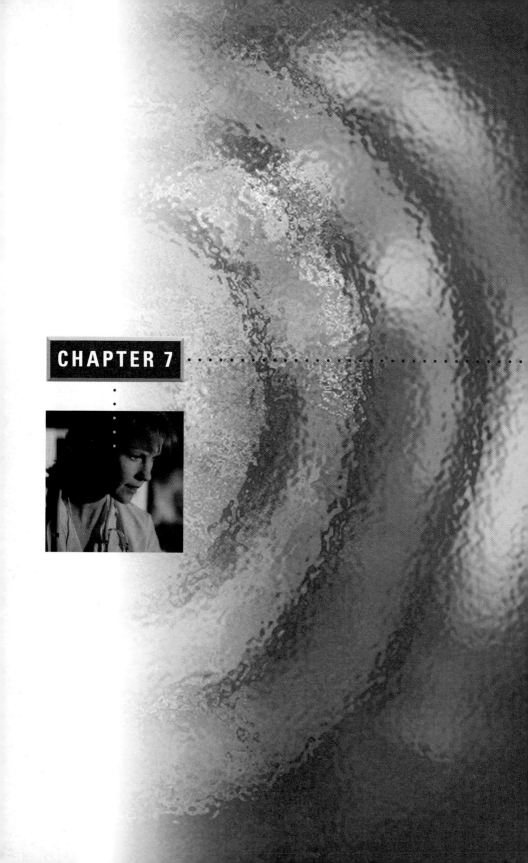

CHAPTER 7

Encouraging Emotional Release Using Humor

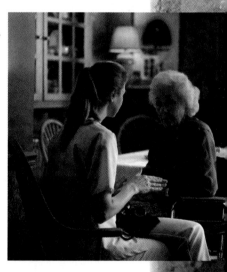

Chapter Objectives

AFTER READING THIS CHAPTER,
YOU WILL BE ABLE TO:

1. Define humor and laughter.
2. Describe the general purposes of humor and laughter.
3. Describe how humor can be used to facilitate therapeutic communication.
4. Describe the benefits of humor in facilitating communication.
5. Distinguish between humor that is therapeutic and nontherapeutic.
6. Describe the physiological effects of humor.
7. Describe the psychological effects of humor.
8. Identify the uses of humor in health care situations by patients and nurses.

UMOR AND LAUGHTER ARE IMPORTANT THERAPEUTIC COMMUNICATION resources that facilitate healing and well-being. They're also effective therapeutic mechanisms for releasing stress-related tensions. A sense of humor, including the ability to laugh with others and to laugh at oneself, has often been linked to good health. This link between happiness and wellness has been known for centuries. For example, during the 18th century, there was a saying that, "The arrival of a single clown has a more healthful impact on the health of a village than that of 20 asses laden with medication."[1] This same idea is also reflected in the more modern version of the expression, "Laughter is the best medicine."

During the late 1970s, Norman Cousins stimulated a scientific interest in the health professions regarding the benefits of humor and laughter during illness. His popular book, *Anatomy of an Illness,* described how 10 minutes of belly laughter rendered him free of pain for 2 hours. He said that humor aided his recovery from ankylosing spondylitis, an immune disorder that causes pain and inflammation of bones and joints.[2] Since then, nurses and other health care researchers have been exploring the therapeutic effects of humor and are finding ways to integrate humor into patient care situations and with each other.[3-6] The use of humor in nursing has become so popular that publications and associations have been developed that are dedicated to promoting therapeutic humor in health care. Some of these informational sources are listed on page 175.

Of course, nurses have always been very serious about providing top-quality nursing care. Nursing education programs and health care institutions expect nurses to take their jobs very seriously, and they do. But many nurses have realized how beneficial humor can be when it is used appropriately. Humor is not appropriate in every situation. It is a tool that needs to be used after careful assessment of the situation and only with knowledge of the emotional state of the patient.

Historically, religious orders and the military were involved with the early nurse training schools. Humor was deemed irreverent, disruptive, and frivolous. Joking and laughter were considered even destructive to a therapeutic relationship and highly unprofessional. Humor was believed to show a lack of concern or that the nurse did not take the patient's problems seriously.

The primary purpose of this chapter is to explore the use of humor in nursing practice. Through therapeutic humor as a communication tool, nurses express openness, warmth, and caring. Therapeutic humor in nursing involves the purposeful use of humor to establish relationships by accelerating the development of trust; relieving anxiety and fear; releasing and defusing anger, hostility, and aggression; and improving patient education.[3-9]

Research suggests that patients expect and appreciate a sense of humor in their nurses and that a sense of humor is regarded as an im-

HUMOR SOURCES

The American Association of Therapeutic Humor
222 S. Meramec, Suite 303
St. Louis, MO 63105
(314) 863-6232
http://ideanurse.com/aath

Journal of Nursing Jocularity Publishing
PO Box 40416
Mesa, AZ 85274
(602)835-6165
http://www.jocularity.com

The Laughter Remedy
45 N. Fullerton, Suite 402
Montclair, NJ 07042
(973) 783-8383
http://www.laughterremedy.com

Humor sources.

portant characteristic of a good nurse.[3,10–12] Humor makes health care providers more human to patients and reduces the distance between the nurse and the patient. Instead of patients having to submit themselves to rigid routines upheld by rigidly authoritarian and even pompous nurses, such as Nurse Ratched in *One Flew over the Cuckoo's Nest,* you communicate to the patient, "I am a friend" and "This is not such a terrible place."[13]

Therapeutic Humor

Therapeutic humor is a form of verbal or nonverbal communication that is used as an adaptive and healthy coping mechanism for reducing stress levels in numerous situations.[3–9] Humor has been generally defined as something that is or has the ability to be funny or amusing and results in smiling or laughter.[7–9] The term *humor* encompasses a number of activities, such as joking, kidding, teasing, clowning, and mimicking. Much of the humor in health settings is spontaneous and specific to a situation. Nurses or patients make witty or humorous comments, producing laughing, smiling, or feelings of amusement. It is typically not formal joke telling.[6-9]

Humor often contains incongruity and surprise that occurs when two ideas are presented in an absurd or impossible situation, as shown in the cartoon on this page. This is a classic cartoon of the nurse waking the patient up to give him a sleeping pill. The first idea is that it is difficult to sleep in a hospital so many people require sleeping pills. The second idea is that patients need to be awakened to give them a pill to sleep, an incongruent and absurd situation.

People express personality through humor. As a characteristic of one's personality, some people have more of a sense of humor and look regularly for the lighter side of a problem, whereas others take things much more seriously. Having a healthy and mature sense of humor means finding enjoyment laughing at the imperfections in ourselves and laughing with others about the imperfect nature of typical

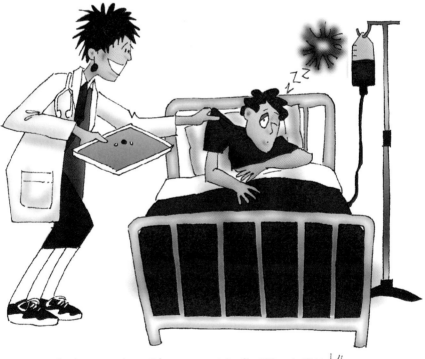

" SIR, IT'S TIME FOR OUR SLEEPING PILL!"

Humor often contains incongruity and surprise when two ideas are presented in an absurd or impossible situation.

daily situations.[14] In addition to laughing with others, a sense of humor involves knowing how to make others laugh.[11] Patients show their sense of humor by joking about their troubles with illness, health insurance, medical bills, diagnostic tests and surgeries, and the care they receive from nurses, doctors, and other health care providers. Likewise, nurses joke about these same things, as well as short staffing, high staff turnover rates, ever-increasing technology, and never-ending paperwork.

Nontherapeutic Humor

Humor is not appropriate when it takes place at the expense of individuals or groups and alienates them. Remember that humor can be used to wound. Jokes that maliciously tease and belittle someone or a group are termed "put-downs." Jokes can be contemptuous or sarcastic, and thus aggressive and hostile expressions of dislike and disdain. For example, children can be merciless as they tease another child who stutters, is obese, or has acne. Ethnic humor or jokes about gender differences can be offensive and indicate prejudice. These jokes are intended as put-downs and insults to express superiority over someone else.[6,15]

In actuality, people who use this type of humor are feeling very insecure. They have low self-esteem and need to build themselves up by putting someone else down. Instead of reducing tension, laughing at someone is insensitive and creates more stressful emotional tension.[1] Nurses need to be very careful never to be insulting with humor. We need to laugh with, but not at, patients and their families.

Humor is not appropriate when a patient is very sick or emotionally distraught. If someone is very fearful, very anxious, very sad, or in great pain, humor will not be appreciated. All of the person's energy is needed to ward off the danger, and the comic effect is lost. The dangerous threat must be controlled before reference to the problem can be enjoyed through humor.[4,5,7-9] When a patient is in a crisis situation, humor results in disgust or horror. For example, consider the patient who was in the recovery room and breathing heavily. The nurse had just assessed his pulse, blood pressure, and ventilatory status and believed that his heavy breathing resulted from anxiety. She said, "Hey buddy, how about controlling that heavy breathing? I've got goose bumps!" The patient was so upset he later stated, "She was so uncaring. I couldn't breathe because it hurt so bad, and she was making jokes!"

What is hilarious to one person can be insulting and tasteless to another. This difference depends on biophysical, psychological, social, cultural, and spiritual states of being. You must first "know your audience" to understand the effect of specific types of humor. You must be sure that the person's emotional and physiological state is stable enough so that you won't be perceived as irritating and uncaring. The criteria for determining the appropriateness of humor is found on page 179.[14]

Physiological Effects of Laughter

Humor often results in smiling and laughter. Why do people feel so good after laughing? The answer to that question requires an understanding of the physiological responses of the body during laughter. People release emotional tensions through laughter. In addition to helping people feel good, laughter can help them heal. Indeed, it can help to prevent them from getting sick in the first place. There are two basic phases of response to laughter: first arousal and then relaxation.

AROUSAL PHASE

During arousal, catecholamines (such as adrenaline) increase. That speeds up our breathing, heart rate, and blood pressure. Depending on how intense the laughter, various groups of muscles contract. When people laugh so hard that they cry, the tears produced contain steroids and other toxins that accumulate under stress.[16] Thus, through secretion of tears, the body regains a healthier biochemical balance.

In addition, the immune system is stimulated into helping the body fight disease.[17-19] During smiling, the zygomaticus major face muscle contracts and stimulates the "master" thymus gland to secrete thymosin, which produces T-cell lymphocytes.[20] These lymphocytes are primary components of the immune defense system, which helps people stay healthy and helps fight disease when they're ill. In addition, laughter increases an antibody found in saliva that prevents upper respiratory infection.[21]

RELAXATION PHASE

People feel terrific after a good laugh. Following arousal and the release of hormones, the body responds automatically by relaxing muscular tensions. In addition, blood pressure and heart rate drop below the prelaughter rate. Laughter promotes breathing patterns that use

Criteria for Determining Appropriateness of Humor in Psychotherapeutic Relationships

Criterion	Determinants
Anxiety level	**Humor** is appropriate when client anxiety is in the mild to moderate range and when the use of humor decreases client anxiety. Humor is inappropriate when client anxiety is in the severe to panic range or when the use of humor increases client anxiety.
Coping style	**Humor** is appropriate when it helps a client cope more effectively, facilitates learning, puts situations in perspective, decreases social distance, and when client cognitive and emotional states permit understanding of and response to humor. Humor is inappropriate when it avoids dealing with problematic situations, masks feelings, increases social distance, and when psychopathology interferes with understanding of or response to humor.
Humor style	**Humor** is appropriate when it conforms with the type of humor and humorist that the client enjoys and when it laughs with people (i.e., laughs at what people do, not at who they are). Humor is inappropriate when it ignores client humor style and when it laughs at people (self-deprecating or other-deprecating humor).

Determining when humor is appropriate in a therapeutic relationship. (Adapted from Pasquali, EA: Learning to laugh: Humor as therapy. Journal of Psychosocial Nursing 28:3, 1990. Reprinted with permission.)

the diaphragm, the opposite of the thoracic breathing that occurs under stress. Diaphragmatic breathing patterns produce respiratory relaxation.[1] The physical state of muscle relaxation can't exist simultaneously with anxiety.[22,23]

Laughter also reduces the perception of pain.[2,11,24,25] The exact mechanism of this effect remains unknown, although it is theorized that laughter stimulates the brain to release endorphins.[7–9] Endorphins are hormones that act as the body's natural pain killers. In addition, endorphins give people happy feelings and sometimes even feelings of euphoria, feelings that are produced when they laugh.

Psychological Effects of Humor

Humor and laughter can lead to beneficial psychological effects as well, especially emotional release. Humor helps us manage stress by enabling the release of nervous tensions. It offers an acceptable outlet for anxiety, fear, and anger. When we are anxious and fearful, we might shake and perspire to release pent-up emotions, characteristics of the flight component of the stress response. However, if we can talk and laugh about our anxiety and fear, we can get therapeutic emotional relief, a much healthier method. Similarly, when we are angry, our bodies seek to get rid of the emotional tension created by the anger. We feel hostile and resentful. We may rant and rave, or we may hit someone or something, the fight component of the stress response, to attain release from our anger. Or we can laugh and talk about our anger to release emotional tensions.[1,4,5]

Without the release of painful emotions, physical, emotional, and mental signs of stress develop, as previously described in Chapter 4. For example, you may feel nauseated (a physical sign), irritable (an emotional sign), and unable to concentrate on what you're supposed to be doing (a mental sign). Excessive tension and a lack of therapeutic emotional release can bring on or aggravate many physical diseases, such as heart disease, diabetes, and ulcers. This reflects the wisdom in the popular phrase "You'll worry yourself sick."

Health care providers who are not skilled in therapeutic communication techniques typically want to quiet an emotionally quickly distraught patient and may medicate patients with tranquilizers and muscle relaxants to produce relaxation in someone who is fearful, anxious, or angry. However, all that the medications will do is dull the sensations of tension. The person becomes sedated and sleepy. Laughter and humor, combined with meaningful verbal conversation, can produce the same beneficial relaxation without the side effects of drugs, such as sedation and drowsiness. The advantage of humor and laughter with verbalization is that the patient maintains the ability to think clearly and solve problems. A nurse who can communicate well can help an emotionally upset patient find ways to deal effectively with the problems underlying the stressful tensions. This is not possible with a drowsy patient.

Please understand that there are many situations in which patients do need to be sedated and sleep, such as before and after many procedures, especially surgery. Patients in these situations do not need humor. They need pain medications and sedatives. By all means, administer these treatments promptly to help get patients past the acute phase of discomfort.

How Patients Use Humor

The humorous messages sent from patients to nurses typically involve situations too painful to communicate directly. Strong negative emotions, such as fear, anger, and loss, may be defused through humor. Thus, humor is often used as an indirect communication between the patient and nurse, and many times, it is used by patients to deliver very serious messages. So listen carefully, then think about and respond to the message behind the humor. If you don't pick up on the message by ignoring a humorous remark, you'll increase the emotional distance between you and the patient, and you'll be ineffective in helping him deal with his situation.

EMOTIONAL SITUATIONS

Patients often express their fears and concerns about body image through jokes. For example, say you're taking vital signs on a patient in the cardiac step-down unit who had cardiac surgery 3 days ago and has been progressing very well. She is a tiny, thin lady who is 78 years old and covered with dark bruises around her chest and leg incisions, around the sites used to obtain blood samples from both arms, and around the area where the central line had been inserted. This is all quite normal and expected after open-heart surgery. The patient is sitting up in bed and, with smiling bright blue eyes, she looks at you and jokingly says, "Just look at me! It looks like someone beat me with a hammer."

You smile at her and say, "We sure do beat patients up around here, no doubt about it!" Then seriously you say, "I'll bet you're wondering if you are ever going to heal from all this. But you know, those black and blue marks are all normal, and they will all go away. Your incisions are also healing nicely, and your blood pressure and heart are doing fine."

Why did the patient make the joking remark? She was asking indirectly, "How am I doing? I look and feel a mess. Will I ever get better from all this?" This remark points to body image disturbance and a need for reassurance. The conversation continued about what the scars would look like after they healed, how long healing usually takes, and how to use makeup and clothing as camouflage.

EMBARRASSING SITUATIONS

Embarrassing situations are numerous in health care settings, including many that involve intimate procedures. Patients commonly joke about bedpans, bathrooms, and enemas to release nervous tension. Sometimes self-ridicule is used by the patient, and we can laugh with the patient. For example, "How is a person with a big butt like mine supposed to fit on that bedpan?" Laughing with the patient would be appropriate. However, what if you had made that comment, "How is someone with a big butt like yours supposed to use this bedpan?" The patient almost certainly would have taken it as an insult. When a patient engages in self-ridicule, then you can laugh—gently—with the patient. But you should never ridicule or insult a patient because that would be laughing at her, not with her.

Patients may be embarrassed to talk about certain subjects and may initiate a topic through humor to determine whether or not it is acceptable to talk about. For example, say you're teaching a 55-year-old male patient with a colostomy how to irrigate and change the bag. In the middle of the irrigation, he laughs and says, "There goes my sex life! I guess I can work on my golf game."

You smile at him and ask seriously, "Do you have some concerns about sex?"

He responds, "My wife has such a weak stomach, she won't even look at this thing on me!"

You continue to let him express his feelings, then you say, "Maybe we can sit down with your wife and discuss this problem together." If you have little experience or knowledge in this area, then you can make a referral to other nurses on your unit or to another health care provider. Nurses are not expected to be marriage counselors unless they have special certification, so it may be very appropriate to assess the situation from the wife's perspective and then make a referral.

UNPLEASANT SITUATIONS

Patients often make jokes about their lack of control over what is being done to them and the hospital routines. They pretend to be in a motel, and they joke about the food and the service they receive. You have undoubtedly seen many such jokes on the fronts of humorous get-well cards. These jokes are actually expressions of the patient's feelings of powerlessness and lack of control. Listen to the message that the patient is really delivering when she jokes. Joke back to her, and then become serious about the topic.

Some patients need to have blood drawn morning, noon, and night. They refer to the blood drawers as the "vampires." As you go to assess your patient, he says jokingly, "Those vampires keep coming to get me. They're sucking all my blood."

You sense that he is actually angry and feels out of control, and you say, "The vampires do come in here a lot, but we need to know the results of all those tests. Do you have some questions about the blood tests?"

The patient says, "I just don't understand why they can't draw it once a day instead of so many times each day." Now you can explain the tests and what they're for, and you can get him involved in what's being done. That should help decrease his feelings of anger and powerlessness.

"HOPELESS" SITUATIONS

Sometimes patients get downhearted and may say to themselves, "This whole situation is hopeless. There's nothing I can do anymore that I like to do. I'll never get better." Tunnel vision and the inability to see options are characteristics of hopelessness and stress. Humor helps alter this narrowed mental perspective and reframe a situation. It also helps to restore a sense of motivation, as comically shown in the cartoon on page 184.

Consider this example. A nurse came to take the pulse of an elderly patient who had just had major surgery. He loved to play bocce ball at the senior citizen club. The patient told the nurse, "I won't be able to play anymore." The nurse tried to reassure him verbally without success. But after taking his pulse, the nurse said, "I can tell you're a bocce ball player from your heartbeat." He looked surprised and then smiled elfishly. "You really think I'll be able to play again?"

In this situation, the patient's depression wasn't so severe that all his affect was frozen. He was able to respond to the warmth and caring the nurse's humor conveyed. The idea is that if we can take a detached view of a situation, we can think more objectively and can begin to problem solve. We can rise above our deficiencies through laughing at ourselves.

AVOIDANCE TACTICS

Sometimes patients use humor to avoid facing problems. In this case, however, humor becomes maladaptive. The patient constantly makes jokes and won't admit or express his true feelings. In this case, humor is used to escape from reality and from confronting and dealing with fears. In other words, humor becomes a way of escaping from difficulties rather than making it easier to deal with difficulties by putting them in a new perspective. In this situation, you'll probably need to

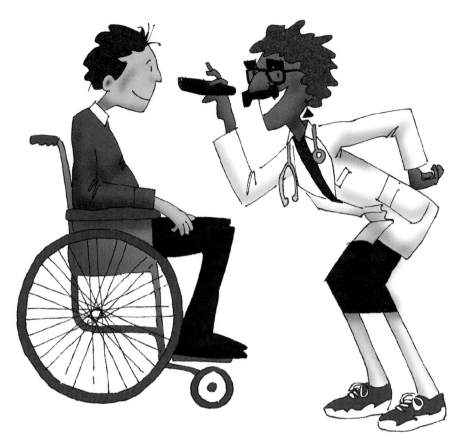

Humor can help alter a patient's narrowed mental perspective and reframe a situation. It also can help to restore a sense of motivation.

confront the patient, help him take a serious look at the situation, and do some problem solving. Problem solving is discussed in Chapter 10.

GENDER DIFFERENCES IN USING HUMOR

Men often use sexually oriented jokes and teasing with the female staff. By doing so, they're asserting the masculinity that's threatened during hospitalization, especially if they perceive themselves to be dependent and powerless. They'll make flirting comments and try to relate as a man to a woman rather than as a patient to an authority figure.

You must realize that the basis for these comments is the threat to his male ego created by the situation. Don't think that you've done anything to encourage him. And remember that if you become embarrassed or uncomfortable, he shows his superiority and control over the situation. Now he's one up on you. Instead of becoming embarrassed or defensive, respond with appropriate banter and then assess the source of the threat the patient is probably feeling.[7-9]

Say, for example, that you're giving the patient a back rub and he says to you, "Honey, how about rubbing down a little lower." You could laugh and playfully hit him on the back and say, "I guess you are feeling well enough to be getting out of here. The sooner the better, I think!" Then say, seriously, "It's very difficult to be in the hospital when there are so many other things I'm sure you'd rather be doing." Now you have recognized the need behind the comment, the threat of dependency and feelings of powerlessness.

How Nurses Use Humor

Above all, remember that humor in nursing is bound to the context of the situation. Under all circumstances, jokes and funny stories must be fitting to the nursing situation and never insulting. It's important to know something about the patient, even to know her well, before you can judge whether or not she'll appreciate the humor you see in a situation.

Usually, if a patient initiates humor by making a humorous remark, you can be almost certain that she'll appreciate your return of humorous remarks or gestures.[11] Joking by nurses often involves playful, light-hearted teasing done with a cheerful attitude. So, as you help a patient into a chair and support him under his arms, you might say, "Shall we dance?" Or if you're taking a patient for a wheelchair ride to physical therapy, you might say, "Step into the limo, ma'am. We're off for our afternoon outing."

MAKING CONTACT

As a nurse, you can't be effective therapeutically until you form a trusting relationship with the patient. Humor is one way of developing that relationship through sharing and expressing thoughts and feelings, including anxieties, fears, and anger. Demonstrating a sense of humor as you meet a patient can also serve to break the ice. When you share laughter with someone, you can quickly make supportive emotional contact.[1,3]

For example, consider the patient who comes in for a clinic visit and you need to ask her to remove all her clothes and put on a flimsy paper gown. She's walking and talking, and so doesn't appear to be highly anxious, fearful, or in pain. Most of us feel embarrassed and uncomfortable without clothes on. So you comment, "Today, just for you, we have a stunning gown to wear during your examination! Isn't it lovely?"

You have demonstrated your sense of humor in an attempt to put the patient at ease and recognize out loud that you know most people are embarrassed by nakedness. You've shown your empathy in a witty manner. The patient responds with a smile and says, "I really hate these gowns, you know. And, the whole thought of a physical worries me."

You've made contact, and the patient told you how she felt. Do you know what to say next? Remember to pick up on the emotion, using empathy. You become serious and look her in the eyes and say, "Oh? What are you worried about?"

MAINTAINING RELATIONSHIPS

As you continue a relationship with a patient, humor helps put the person at ease and may increase cooperation with what you ask him to do. When you need to give an injection, for example, you might say, "I have a soft and little needle for you because you're one of my favorite patients. I promise only a tiny pinch. Let's get this done. I'll be very quick about it." You are implying, "Relax, this isn't so terrible. You can trust me."

Or before sending a patient to surgery, you could jest, "Have a nice trip. We'll keep your bed warm for you, and we'll see you in a little bit." All patients going off to surgery are nervous about it. Some patients just show it more than others. Humor keeps that anxiety in check. You give a patient confidence by these remarks. You imply that things are going fine and that everything is under control and proceeding according to routine.

EMOTIONAL STABILITY

You can also use humor with other nurses to distance yourself from pain and suffering. In fact, nurses commonly use a macabre form of humor that people outside of nursing may not find funny in the least. Here's an example. The evening intensive care unit (ICU) nurses were sitting at the conference table and had just finished hearing the day shift's patient report. One of the night nurses had called in sick, and there was no one to replace her. It was going to be a long evening without enough staff and very busy. Eight of 11 patients in the medical ICU were on ventilators, unconscious, and in critical condition. One remarked to the others, "We're working in a vegetable garden tonight." The others laughed, and another nurse said, "Well, everyone grab your shovels and buckets, and let's get to work. We're good. We'll get through it." Everyone laughed again.

These nurses were under great stress and actually wondering how they were going to make it through the evening. How were they going to take care of these very ill people? They probably would hardly get more than a few minutes break all night. The joking relieved the frustration by detaching them from the situation. However, it's a good thing that no family members were around to here this grim humor. It would have been very disturbing to hear their loved one on a ventilator referred to as a vegetable. Freud described this as gallows humor, in which one laughs at death and tragedy to help cope with a morbid situation.[26–29]

PATIENT EDUCATION

Humor stimulates us physically and mentally, and its use may make patients more receptive to information and increase their willingness to explore and analyze new ideas.[28] Humor can be used to strengthen major points or basic ideas that must be conveyed to the patient during teaching.[15] Humorous information can often be remembered longer and more easily than information presented in a formal manner. Humor can include funny definitions of key terms, puns, exaggerations, and understatements. Cartoons can help patients remember and recall what they were taught about postoperative exercises.[29] Humorous and light analogies, anecdotes, and parables can help teach family planning and health concepts.[21]

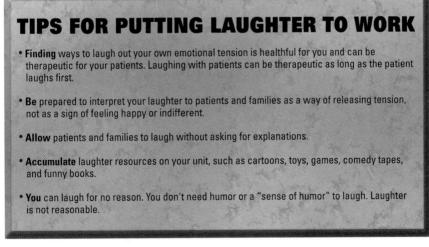

TIPS FOR PUTTING LAUGHTER TO WORK

- **Finding** ways to laugh out your own emotional tension is healthful for you and can be therapeutic for your patients. Laughing with patients can be therapeutic as long as the patient laughs first.

- **Be** prepared to interpret your laughter to patients and families as a way of releasing tension, not as a sign of feeling happy or indifferent.

- **Allow** patients and families to laugh without asking for explanations.

- **Accumulate** laughter resources on your unit, such as cartoons, toys, games, comedy tapes, and funny books.

- **You** can laugh for no reason. You don't need humor or a "sense of humor" to laugh. Laughter is not reasonable.

Tips for putting laughter to work. (Adapted from Dugan, DO: Laughter and tears: Best medicine for stress. Nursing Forum 24:1, 1989. Reprinted with permission.)

For example, you might write humorous expressions related to a class topic on nametags and then have each patient choose a nametag at the beginning of class. Each patient can then introduce himself and explain why he chose the humorous expression he did.[30] These name tags can be used as ice breakers to help establish a warm and congenial environment, to set the tone for the class, and to put the patients at ease. The use of humor in patient education is described further in Chapter 9, which is devoted to communication during patient education.

Now You've Blown It: Making a Mistake with Humor

What happens if you're trying to be humorous and a patient becomes offended by misinterpreting the intent of your humor? The patient is upset and distressed. You must quickly become serious and apologize, saying, "I'm sorry. This is really a serious concern and I shouldn't have tried to be humorous about it." If the patient believes that you're truly interested in her welfare, the blunder will be forgiven.

SUMMARY   Humor and laughter are cost-effective and time-effective health promotion tools. Nurses are finding ways to use humor and laughter as a means to communicate effectively with patients. Like other skills, it must be practiced if it is to become part of your therapeutic communication techniques. You must expand your sense of humor by developing an attitude that allows you to see the absurdities in situations, others, and especially, in yourself.

Humor involves either situational dilemmas or points out human weaknesses we can all relate to. When you can see the absurdity and laugh at it, you can distance yourself from problems that threaten you. Humor is an effective coping mechanism when used to reframe reality, diminish negative feelings, and experience relief. As depicted on page 187, nurses need to find ways to put laughter to work for them in patient care situations.[1]

However, what is considered funny and amusing to one person may be insulting, tasteless, embarrassing, or emotionally painful to another. It is important never to be insulting with humor and to assess each patient carefully for physical and emotional discomforts before trying to use humor.

Humor is not a cure-all. Nurses are using humor as a specific therapeutic communication intervention to help them in working with patients and families. It is important to note that humor is only one tool, one mechanism for coping and one teaching methodology. There are many, many others.

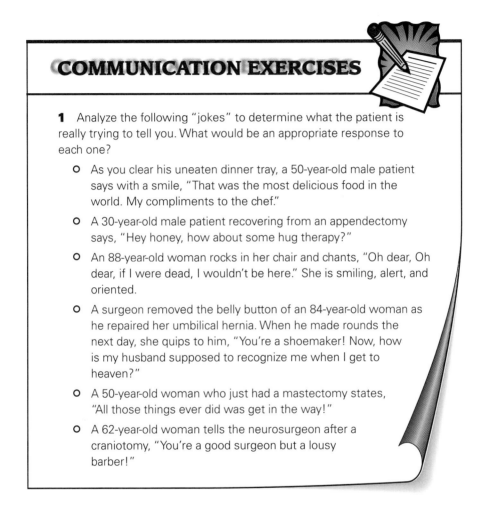

COMMUNICATION EXERCISES

1 Analyze the following "jokes" to determine what the patient is really trying to tell you. What would be an appropriate response to each one?

- As you clear his uneaten dinner tray, a 50-year-old male patient says with a smile, "That was the most delicious food in the world. My compliments to the chef."

- A 30-year-old male patient recovering from an appendectomy says, "Hey honey, how about some hug therapy?"

- An 88-year-old woman rocks in her chair and chants, "Oh dear, Oh dear, if I were dead, I wouldn't be here." She is smiling, alert, and oriented.

- A surgeon removed the belly button of an 84-year-old woman as he repaired her umbilical hernia. When he made rounds the next day, she quips to him, "You're a shoemaker! Now, how is my husband supposed to recognize me when I get to heaven?"

- A 50-year-old woman who just had a mastectomy states, "All those things ever did was get in the way!"

- A 62-year-old woman tells the neurosurgeon after a craniotomy, "You're a good surgeon but a lousy barber!"

References

1. Dugan, DO: Laughter and tears: Best medicine for stress. Nursing Forum *24*:18, 1989.
2. Cousins, N: The Anatomy of an Illness. Norton, New York, 1979.
3. Fosbinder, D: Patient perceptions of nursing care: An emerging theory of interpersonal competence. Journal of Advanced Nursing *20*:1085, 1994.
4. McGhee, P: Rx: Laughter. RN *98*:50, 1998.

5. McGhee, P: Health, Healing, and the Amuse System. Kendall/Hunt, Dubuque, IA, 1996.
6. Fonnesbeck, BG: Are you kidding? Nursing98 28(3):64, 1998.
7. Robinson, V: Humor and health. In McGhee, PE, and Goldstein, JH (eds): Handbook of Humor Research, Vol. 2. Applied Studies. Springer-Verlag, New York, 1983, p 109.
8. Robinson, VM: Humor and the Health Professions, ed 2. Slack Incorporated, Thorofare, NJ, 1977.
9. Robinson, V: Humor in nursing. In Carlson, C, and Blackwell, B (eds): Behavioral Concepts and Nursing Intervention, ed 2. J. B. Lippincott, Philadelphia, 1978.
10. Schmitt, N: Patients' perception of laughter in a rehabilitation hospital. Rehabilitation Nursing 15(3):143, 1990.
11. Astedt-Kurki, P: Humour in nursing care. Journal of Advanced Nursing 20:183,1994.
12. Astedt-Kurki, P, and Haggman-Laitila, A. Good nursing practice as perceived by clients: A starting point to the development of professional nursing. Journal of Advanced Nursing 17: 1195, 1992.
13. Kesey, K: One Flew Over the Cuckoo's Nest: A Novel. Penguin Books, New York, 1962.
14. Morreall, J: Taking Laughter Seriously. State University of New York Press, Albany, New York, 1983.
15. Pasquali, EA: Learning to laugh: Humor as therapy. Journal of Psychosocial Nursing 28:31,1990.
16. Ruxton, JP: Humor intervention deserves our attention. Holistic Nursing Practice 2:54,1988.
17. Berk, LS, and Tan, SA: Immune system changes during humor associated with laughter. Clinical Research 39:124A, 1991.
18. Berk, LS, Tan, SA, and Fry, W: Eustress of humor-associated laughter modulates specific immune system components. Annals of Behavioral Medicine 15(Suppl):S111, 1993.
19. Berk, LS, and Tan, SA: A positive emotion, the eustress of mirthful laughter modulates the immune system lymphokine interferon-gamma. Psychoneuroimmunology Research Society Annual Meetings, April (abstract supplement) 5:A1, 1995.
20. Mazer, E: 10 sure-fire stress releasers. Prevention 34:104,1989.
21. Diamond, J: Your Body Doesn't Lie. Warner, New York, 1979.
22. Flavier, JM: The lessons of laughter. World Health Forum 11:412, 1990.
23. Samra, C: A time to laugh. Journal of Christian Nursing 3:17, 1985.
24. Siegel, B: Love, Medicine and Miracles. Harper & Row: New York, 1986.
25. Nevo, O, Keinan, G, and Teshimousky-Ardit, M: Humor and pain tolerance. International Journal of Humor Research 6:71, 1993.
26. Williams, H: Humour and healing. Therapeutic effects in geriatrics. Gerontion 1:14,1986.
27. Freud, S: Humor. International Journal of Psychoanalysis 9:1, 1928.
28. Freud, S: Jokes and their relationship to the unconscious. In Strachey, J (ed): The Complete Psychological Works of Sigmund Freud, Vol 8. Hogarth Press: London, 1961.
29. Parfitt, JM: Humorous preoperative teaching. AORN Journal 52:114, 1990.
30. White, LA, and Lewis, DJ: Humor: A teaching strategy to promote learning. Journal of Nursing Staff Development 3:60,1990.

Encouraging Emotional Release Through Tears

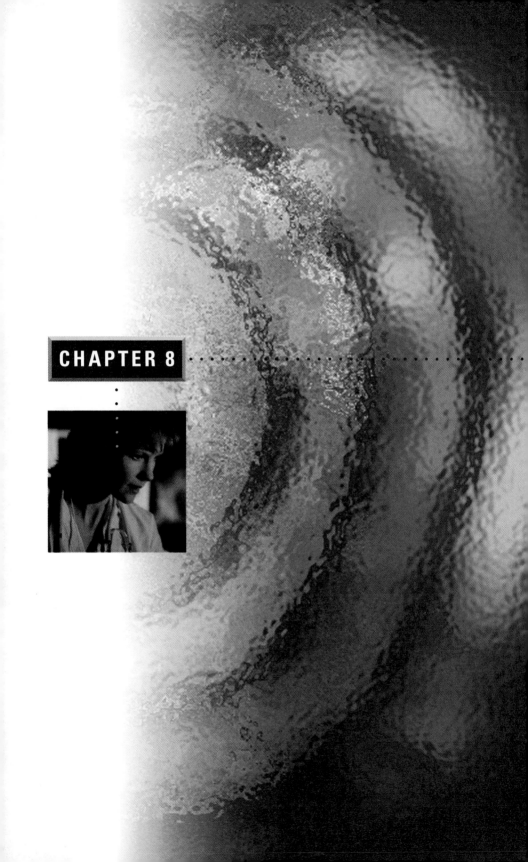

CHAPTER 8

Encouraging Emotional Release Through Tears

. . . .

Chapter Objectives

AFTER READING THIS CHAPTER,
YOU WILL BE ABLE TO:

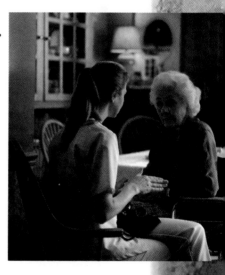

1. Describe how tears can be used to promote emotional healing after loss, grief, fear, frustration, and anger.

2. Compare how tears and crying can be therapeutic versus how they can be used to manipulate and control.

3. Describe the physiological processes that occur with the release of tears.

4. Describe the relationships of anger, fear, and sadness with tears.

5. Identify appropriate and inappropriate nursing responses when a patient or family member cries.

6. Describe gender differences in emotional release using tears.

TEARS AND CRYING ARE A VERY IMPORTANT THERAPEUTIC RESOURCE THAT you can use to facilitate healing and well-being. That's because nurses routinely help patients and families cope with anger, fear, and losses associated with illness and its treatment. The stress-related emotional tensions caused by anger, fear, sadness, and loss can be effectively released through crying and tears. However, providing emotional support to a crying patient or family member is a difficult challenge for many nurses. The purpose of this chapter is to explore the purposes of crying and tears, and appropriate nursing responses when a patient or family member cries.

Nontherapeutic Responses to Crying

Many nurses feel uncomfortable when a patient cries. Naturally, it's easy for nurses to feel bad about a patient's unpleasant situation and become upset and anxious themselves when the patient cries. So, to reduce their own feelings of discomfort, these nurses may want to quickly quiet the patient or family member. To do so, they may minimize the patient's cause for crying or express disapproval of the crying. Comments include, "There's no need to cry. You're doing fine." or "Let's stop crying now." By quieting the patient, the nurse spares herself the need to address her own emotional turmoil as well as that of the patient. Other responses intended to quiet a patient and bury emotions and problems include such comments as, "Get hold of yourself" (advice), "Think positive" (more advice), "Think of your family" (guilt), "I promise that everything will be fine" (false reassurance), or "You shouldn't feel that way" (judgmental).

People who prefer to avoid the emotions that result in crying may also choose certain expressions to convey condolences after the death of a loved one. These expressions deny the importance of the grief or imply that the person has no right to grieve for a loss. These comments include, "You must be strong," which implies that only weak people show grief; "You must be a man about this," which implies that men and boys shouldn't cry or grieve; and "It's time to get on with your life," which implies that grieving should consume a certain amount of time, after which the person no longer has a right to grieve.

If you can hear yourself making any of these statements, then you don't understand—and aren't trying to understand—the feelings of people who are crying. Your best course of action is to erase these comments permanently from your list of appropriate things to say when someone is crying, or at any other time! These remarks might help you feel better, but they aren't therapeutic and they'll block further expression of emotions. These blocks were discussed in Chapter 4. In addition, as previously discussed, you should never offer false hope or make promises you can't keep.

Sometimes, if patients become too upset in a health care provider's opinion, crying and tears may be viewed as a problem to be treated with drugs. Instead of allowing the release of painful emotions and the examination of underlying emotional pain, we can subdue and control emotional expression by administering tranquilizing medications to sedate and numb emotional pain. Always remember that drugs may provide an easy way to quiet a person and perhaps get them to sleep, but drugs can never recognize or resolve real problems.

A "Good" Cry

Weeping helps a person feel better because tears can reduce perceived emotional pain levels and can actually create pleasant sensations. Tears are therapeutic because they are cathartic coping mechanisms to help resolve feelings of loss, grief, fear, frustration, and anger. There are chemicals in tears that help to reduce stress.[1] If we shut off the tears and ignore the emotional pain, the tensions are not released and the waste chemicals excreted in tears remain trapped in the body.

By releasing stress-related tensions and hormones, crying produces a relaxation response. Initially, tears stimulate the sympathetic nervous system, causing the release of catecholamines that increase blood pressure and heart rate. This arousal is followed by a parasympathetic response that generates a state of systemic relaxation. Sobbing leads to respiratory relaxation by producing diaphragmatic breathing patterns instead of the thoracic tension-producing breathing pattern associated with the fight-or-flight response. We feel "pleasantly drained" after a good long cry.[2]

Loss, Sadness, and Grief

With unresolved loss and grief, sadness turns into depression—emotional depression and also physiological depression of the immune system. Thus, affected people are more susceptible to colds and flu, and they can have symptoms of emotional depression and stress, such as fatigue, headaches, and backaches.[3] Over a period of time, classic signs of the stress response arise, as described in Chapter 4.

Tears are shed when tensions accompany disappointment and sadness. We feel a sense of loss. Tensions associated with loss include such symptoms as tightness in the chest, choking, shortness of breath, sighing, empty feelings in the stomach, and feelings of weakness.[4] These feelings are very distressing. Tears must flow if the loss is to be resolved and the tensions are to be released.

People cry for many specific reasons, but there always is some form of loss involved when a person cries. All people have experienced loss as they go through each stage of their lives. If people can learn to recognize and grieve appropriately for small losses, they'll be better prepared to deal with the big losses that inevitably occur in all lives.[5] Unexpressed grief over loss negatively effects behavior and emotional well-being. People become unable to function in their personal lives or their jobs.

Many people cry at weddings, graduations, or when moving to a newer and bigger home, even though these are supposedly happy events. You may be confused as to why some people feel sad or depressed at these happy events. The sadness is caused by the losses that will result at an otherwise happy event.

Learning how to deal with loss may be one of life's most difficult and most important lessons. There are many types of losses that people grieve about throughout life. For example, a person feels very bad about losing a ring that was given to her by her great-grandmother and grieves for the loss of the object. A person grieves for the loss of a special relationship, hopes, and dreams when a marriage ends in divorce. If a job is lost, the person grieves for its loss as well as the loss of income. During an illness, the person may grieve for the loss of body image, such as with mastectomy. Of course, people grieve the loss when a loved one dies. Depending on the loss and the meaning of the loss to the individual, some people may also experience a loss of security, self-esteem, their belief system, or their faith.

Losses occur throughout the life span. Each loss involves pain that we must learn to cope with to maintain emotional and physical health. It is especially important for health care providers to understand the significance of loss, typical reactions to loss, and how to be supportive of patients and families who are grieving a loss.

Before you can help others, it is important to recognize and acknowledge your own vulnerability to loss and pain. You must acknowledge that you can never be in total control of your life, and that some events are beyond your control. Once you make this acknowledgment, it's easier to deal with the fear, guilt, and anger caused by a loss over which you had no control. You must also acknowledge your own mortality, and that life as you know it on earth will end someday.

Gains and Losses Throughout Growth and Development

Everyone's life involves a series of changes, some of them gains and some of them losses. You've probably heard the expression "You've got to take the good along with the bad." Don't make that statement to someone who is in the grieving process because it wouldn't be therapeutic. However, there is some truth to the statement. Bad things happen to everyone. Losses are part of everyone's life, and we must learn to deal with bad things. At each stage of growth and development, people must learn to recognize their feelings and then work through the emotions as they react to the losses. Nurses must recognize that it takes time to grieve and that everyone has the right to grieve for their losses, big and small. Accepting the joy and coping with the pain leads to a full life.

Nursing students take psychology courses on healthy emotional growth and development throughout the life span. The students must understand the typical struggles of psychological growth and development, and do an assessment to evaluate gains and losses of patients and families before their present health situation. Once you understand what was going on in their lives before a loss, you have the basis for showing empathy and understanding the meaning of sickness or death to patients and family members. You can become tolerant and accepting of all kinds of emotional expression, and you can encourage patients and families to express themselves in whatever ways they feel comfortable.

BIRTH AND INFANCY

With a healthy pregnancy and delivery of a healthy baby, the birth experience is a very happy event. However, the birth is the end of pregnancy. The one-time attachment between the mother and fetus is lost. In addition, mothers may also feel blue because the attention they received during pregnancy is now focused on the baby. Plus, their bodies will never be the same, and some mothers feel overwhelmed at how much work is needed to get back in shape.

If the mother breastfeeds, she can form a special bond with the infant. However, weaning is a loss because both mother and baby no longer have this special relationship. The developmental task of infancy is learning to trust others to meet their basic human needs for comfort, food, love and security.[6,7]

CHILDHOOD

During early childhood, any separation from the parents is a loss. The child does not know that the parents will return but eventually gains an understanding that they can love and trust other people besides their parents. As the child grows, he becomes increasingly independent. Entering preschool and kindergarten is exciting and frightening because the child loses the security of home, although he gains new experiences, friends, and teachers.

Throughout his school life, the child is promoted and loses a familiar teacher and gains a new one. Friendships break up because interests change, classmates move, or the child himself may move and experience numerous losses.[6,7]

ADOLESCENCE

Promotions to middle school and high school mean giving up many childhood things to become an adolescent. Developmental tasks include becoming autonomous from parents, taking the initiative to try new things, and becoming industrious and winning recognition for their achievements at school and in extracurricular activities.

Adolescent life events include establishing relationships with members of the opposite sex, getting a job, and graduating. When a relationship ends, both teens may feel intense loss, even if the relationship wasn't sexual and they both agreed to split up. A job is a significant gain of a new role and an income. If a job is terminated, however, the role and income are lost. Graduation is a happy event, but it results in the breaking up of many relationships and, in many cases, leaving home. The relatively carefree life of childhood and adolescence ends forever as the adolescent takes on adult responsibilities. The major developmental task is to develop a sense of identity and decide on a career.[6,7]

YOUNG ADULTHOOD

The young adult struggles for financial independence, starts a career, forms close sexual relationships, starts a family, and sets up a home. Each event has the potential for satisfaction and happiness but also has the potential for loss. These losses could come from being fired;

from being divorced; from sustaining property damage through fire, theft, flood, or other disaster; from moving and the consequent loss of friends and their support; and from the death of friends or family members. The major developmental task of young adulthood is to develop intimacy in relationships, develop a career, and start a family.[6,7]

MIDDLE AGE

During the middle adult years, many people find enjoyment in the fruits of their labors. However, the gains and losses of life continue. Sometimes a promotion means salary and prestige but a loss of free time. Expenses peak as children reach college age. A real sense of loss occurs as children leave home to attend school, marry, or get their own apartments. Parents welcome the growing independence of their children, but they experience a loss that the children no longer need them in the same ways. The parent-child relationship changes to an adult-adult relationship. As the last child leaves home, many parents—especially mothers—experience a well-known depressive event called the "empty nest syndrome." Although they are joyful at a child's independence, parents miss having the child around as much, and the daily relationship with the child must change. Also, the role of a parent with children to raise is gone forever.

Sometimes in middle adulthood, people realize that they may not be able to achieve all the goals they aspired to in their youth. They experience a sense of loss. At some point, a person in middle age faces the realization of lost youth. He sees changes in body proportions, wrinkles, vision changes, gray hair, sometimes baldness, and the loss of physical stamina. Women must adapt to menopause and the loss of fertility. Although a man's sexual function can continue into his 80s, temporary dysfunction may become more evident at middle age and may be traumatic.

Many middle-aged adults adapt and accept the effects of time. However, others experience a midlife crisis and set out to prove that they are still young. Divorces occur as one partner seeks out younger companions. Middle age is especially difficult for people who emphasize youth and sex appeal as a way of life. A major task of middle adults is generativity, which involves guiding the next generation through home, work, and community activities.[6,7]

LATE ADULT LIFE

In late adulthood, losses far outnumber gains. There is continued physical decline in all organ systems; the most noticeable include visual and hearing losses, difficulties with mobility, and loss of memory.

Friends and family members are lost through moving and death. Retirement can be viewed as a significant loss of productive activity, loss of income, and loss of relationships.

When a person is deemed no longer able to drive or no longer able to live alone, there is a loss of independence, which most elderly people fear keenly. Moving to a retirement home or nursing home involves the loss of one's home and all that was familiar in that environment. After major losses, such as retirement or movement to a nursing home, many people experience a significant decline in health.

In preparation for death, even though life has been very productive and full, elderly people fear losing their minds, losing control of their lives, becoming a burden, and having more pain than they can bear. The primary task of the older adult is to develop a sense of ego integrity, in which the person can look back on life with a sense of satisfaction with life and acceptance of impending death.[6,7]

Sickness and Death Throughout Life

Now imagine what happens when someone at any stage of life becomes seriously ill (or dies). The patient and family have been picked up out of the typical daily struggles and thrown into a crisis. The meaning and response to the crisis vary with the growth and development of the person and family before the crisis. The usual growth and development tasks are interrupted.

A typical nursing diagnosis at this time is "Altered roles and relationships as a result of illness." The resulting nursing care plan will be focused on how to help patients and families adjust to altered roles and relationships, and especially helping patients and families to grieve their losses.

GRIEF

The word grief involves a process that all people experience, usually after the death of a loved one or another significant loss. Anticipatory grief refers to the type of grief that occurs before an actual loss, usually during a terminal illness.

Grief is an intense and painful emotional state. Grief work involves the process of working through the emotional reaction to loss and reorganizing lifestyles to accommodate the loss. The emotional reaction may last for an extended period. After the loss of a pet, a person may experience 20 hours of crying. The loss of a spouse, parent, child, or close friend may result in 200 or even 300 hours of crying. Tears are common even years after the loss of someone who has been very close.[2]

Tears release the sadness, anger, hate, and guilt commonly present with anticipatory grieving and grief. Recurrent dreams and memories make it difficult to concentrate or to sleep. In early grief, talking through tears about the final days with the deceased and reviewing the good and the bad memories can be therapeutic.

A major loss means that the person must modify her belief system to fit a new reality. The new reality means that the person must restructure and rebuild her life without the loved one who died. In a grief reaction to significant loss, a person might say, "I just don't know what to believe in any more." The person must be able to work through the feelings and then let go of the past when she's ready.

Loss requires a person to say good-bye to someone who has been a very important part of her life. It doesn't mean, however, that she should forget the person or diminish the value of the person or object that was lost. It means closing the door on what was lost and opening a new door to a new life without the lost person. The person must also believe that she can learn to cope with whatever loss she may experience. Triumph over the loss means the person still sees a purpose in living life and becomes actively involved in meaningful activities once more.[5,8]

Old relationships are modified, and new ones are formed. As time passes, feelings of sadness turn to loneliness and then to feelings of hopefulness. The focus is less on the loss and more on the changes needed to adjust. Successful resolution of the loss gives the survivor a greater understanding of life, with greater compassion for suffering and a higher sensitivity to the needs of others.

Grief work

A grieving person should be allowed to choose whether he wants to be around others and participate in activities. The person may need a period of denial and withdrawal. However, too long a period of denial and withdrawal may lead to hyperactivity, hostility, depression, changes in relationships with others, and overall decreased ability to function. Therefore, anyone who has suffered a loss should be encouraged to grieve and continue to have the emotional support of family and friends until they are done grieving. Grieving for the death of a loved one who was very close may extend over at least a year but up to a period of 3 years. Throughout these years, certain people, objects, events, and special occasions evoke memories of the deceased, bringing on feelings of sadness and depression, with resultant tears to relieve the feelings.[5,6,8]

FRUSTRATION AND ANGER

Have you ever been around someone who is so frustrated that he is in tears? The person may be angry about a situation he cannot seem to resolve, or is trying very hard to do something but without success. Frustrations and anger commonly occur in everyday situations, as well as during times of big loss. Perhaps the person is feeling embarrassed and humiliated. In these situations, the person feels a sense of loss because he hasn't lived up to his own self-expectations. His self-esteem has been delivered a blow, and he's unhappy with himself; crying helps relieve the tension.

FEAR AND PAIN

Sometimes people cry because they are frightened. They don't know if an outcome will be good or not, or if they'll be able to cope with a situation. For example, a patient may be afraid of the outcomes of diagnostic testing. A patient who earlier had computed tomographic (CT) scan may cry and say, "I'm afraid the tests will show I have cancer." The person fears the changes that may occur in his lifestyle if the diagnosis of cancer is confirmed. He also fears death.

Small children often cry on the way to surgery because they're afraid of being separated from their parents. Even older children may be afraid to be without their parents, who have always protected them and made them feel safe and secure. Crying in adults and children is therapeutic because it releases the tensions associated with their fears.

People also cry when they are in pain, mainly because the pain and what the pain means frightens them. Pain means that something is wrong, and something wrong means that they can no longer do what they would rather be doing. Thus, in a sense, pain is also a loss: the loss of the ability to do what one would rather be doing. People are afraid of pain, especially if they don't know how to manage it, if they don't know what's causing it, and if they don't know how much damage has been done to their body to cause the pain.

Gender Differences in Shedding Tears

Gender differences in communication are the focus of Chapter 2. This section further expands the specific concept of gender and crying. Women commonly vent their tensions, anger, and frustrations by crying. Men do so more often by yelling and shouting. There is cultural pressure for men not to cry because it is not manly and they will be labeled a sissy or a crybaby.[1] This is clearly delineated in the expression "You're a big boy. Big boys don't cry." In contrast, girls are permitted to cry and express themselves. Thus, male and female children have been culturally conditioned to respond differently. Always keep in mind that men are probably experiencing just as much emotional turmoil as women, even though they do not cry as readily.

Men generally tend not to open up as much as women. They tend to hold their feelings inside and reveal less personal information when they are emotionally overwhelmed and will tend to stifle their tears. However, men are beginning to recognize the importance of crying in releasing pent-up emotions and dealing with stress. Men and boys are being encouraged to show their emotions and not to be afraid to let out tears of true emotion.[1] Men are realizing that crying shows sensitivity and is acceptable when one is touched or emotionally moved.

For example, General H. Norman Schwarzkopf wept when he relinquished his command after winning the Persian Gulf War. He openly wiped away tears several times during his speech. This honest and open display of emotion said much about him and endeared him even more deeply to many people. It's also healthier to release tensions through tears in close relationships. Tears can break down barriers and build stronger bonds in relationships.[1]

However, tears can also be used as weapons. During conflict, tears can be manipulative and have a controlling intent. As a result of manipulation, all involved can feel increased frustration, tension, and alienation.[2] For example, suppose you don't want to do something for someone, and as a result, she begins to cry. Then you feel guilty, selfish, and sorry for her. You agree to do what she wants, but at the same time, you feel resentful toward her because you feel manipulated and controlled. You have assumed the role of the Placater. You need to use assertive and responsive communication to manage a situation when the intent of a person's tears is to manipulate and control. Assertive and responsive communication is the focus of Chapter 5.

It is interesting to note that women in all societies cry more than men, possibly because of hormonal differences between the genders. Women secrete 30 times more of the hormone prolactin than men do. Prolactin is involved chemically with secretions of milk and tears. It is believed that women cry more than men do because of their increased prolactin levels.[2]

Therapeutic Responses to Crying

Let's assume that you're making rounds and you find an elderly woman patient sitting in bed with tears in her eyes and on her cheeks.

You have no idea what could be the matter. Without any other information to go on, you estimate at this point that she is mildly upset.

The basic empathic approach is *always* to deal with the emotion first. Let the emotion out, and let it be recognized. So you say, "I can see that you're upset," and offer her a tissue. Next, sit down so you're on the same level with the patient. Make eye contact and prepare to use active listening skills. Also use touch, such as a hug or a hand on the patient's hand or arm as you say, "What's going on?" or "What are these tears about?" Follow that with a smile and, "I'm a good listener."

As the patient speaks, nod and use facilitators, such as restatement and clarification, to get a very clear picture of the patient's view of her situation. Resist all temptation to interrupt, give advice, change the subject, or give a pep talk. Listen as she tells you through her tears that she has a son who doesn't have time to come and see her as often as she'd like. She explains that he is working and has his own family now, and that she misses him and his family. Her husband died a year ago as well, and she misses him, too. She adds, "I'm just sitting here feeling blue."

To respond with empathy, say something like, "I can see you miss them, and you're probably feeling a bit lonely." Then encourage her to talk about her son or her husband. For example, you could say, "When was the last time you saw your son or his family?" or "How long were you married?" You are showing your interest in her situation by asking these questions.

Although you can do nothing to change the patient's situation, you have helped her to feel better by allowing her to release emotions through tears and words. The patient also recognizes that you care about her enough to take a few minutes to listen to her situation and empathize with her.

In the above-mentioned example, the patient was able to talk though the tears. What about a person who rages and weeps at the same time? Consider, for example, a 30-year-old woman who had been married for 5 years. She was in the gynecology clinic when she got the news that she had gonorrhea. She was waiting in the examining room, where the nurse was supposed to teach her about the disease, its transmission, its prevention, and the importance of obtaining information about her sexual partners. Just as the nurse began teaching, the patient flew into a rage and shouted, "How could he do this to me?" She was crying and cursing at the same time. She threw her purse onto the floor, kicked it across the room, and paced back and forth as she cursed and cried.

The nurse handed her two pillows from the examination table and said, "Here, you can throw these." She threw one and pounded on the other one. The nurse stood up and remained calm as the patient raged. In this case, it was better not to speak at that point, to show acceptance of the behavior, and to wait for the patient to regain control.

Silence is a way of showing acceptance while someone is blowing off steam. Silence also helps a patient collect her thoughts.

Then the patient sat down in a chair and began to sob. The nurse sat in a chair next to her, took her hand, and offered tissue. "I know you're hurting," she said, recognizing verbally the pain the woman was feeling over her husband's betrayal. The patient was able to talk more calmly but was still crying, "I'm sorry I've behaved so badly. I just don't know what I'm supposed to do now." The nurse says, "I'm here for you and we can figure out together what you can do now."

When someone is extremely upset and in great emotional pain, the therapeutic response is to put the patient's own cathartic release mechanisms to work for them. Let the person beat on a pillow or throw something, as long as she isn't hurting herself by the catharsis. Simply allow her to rage and weep, and be open and accepting so that the patient can release emotional tension. There's no use trying to talk with the person during a rage because words aren't enough to alleviate deep feelings of discomfort and severe emotional pain. Once the release has been obtained, the patient will be calmer and able to talk. With your assistance and possibly that of other health care professionals, she can begin to think about the problem and what to do next.

Helping Families Know What To Do When a Loved One is Dying

It's very therapeutic for family members to share in the dying process, for both the patient and the family. Many dying patients say that their greatest fear is dying alone. They want family with them. For survivors, being with the patient in the final moments is therapeutic as well and will facilitate the grief process. A common belief is that witnessing a death or viewing a body immediately after death will be too traumatic. In actuality, this belief inhibits the grief process.

Hospitals can be very intimidating, and the family may want to stay out of the way. However, they may miss the final opportunity to be with the dying person. Encourage close family members to stay with the patient and to talk and touch as much as possible throughout the dying process, even if the patient is comatose. In hospital settings, let the family provide as much care for the family member as they would like, such as bathing or shaving the patient. As an alternative, a terminally ill person may join a hospice program that provides palliative care throughout the dying process. The patient may be able to die at home if he so chooses.

The best thing we can do as health care providers is to communicate acceptance. Use active listening and encourage patients to express their feelings. Encourage patients to work though an impending loss at their own speed. Check in on the patient and family and let them know you are available. Offer food and drink to the family. Do all you can to provide comfort measures, and allow the patient as many choices as possible. As appropriate, offer to call the hospital chaplain or a pastor, priest, rabbi, or other spiritual leader of the patient's choice. Social workers can also help families deal with grief and will know which community resources to seek out.

Nurses Cry, Too

As a nurse, you may identify with situations that don't involve you personally. You'll feel sorry for patients and families, and you'll identify with them. You'll become emotionally involved, and you'll cry.

Even when people aren't real, you may find yourself crying. For example, think of a sad movie that made you cry. You became tied to the characters in the movie and felt a sense of acute loss and grief at the end of the movie. Most of the people in the theater were crying, too, for the same reason. Or perhaps you see a very sad story on the news, such as the Oklahoma bombing. It's natural to become teary as you see the suffering of victims being carried from the scene and the distraught relatives of those who died. Many people grieve with the family members of those who were injured and died, and can only imagine the loss they must be feeling.

When caring for patients and families, you'll become close to them and experience grief along with them. You'll cry—and should cry—to release the tensions associated with that grief. For example,

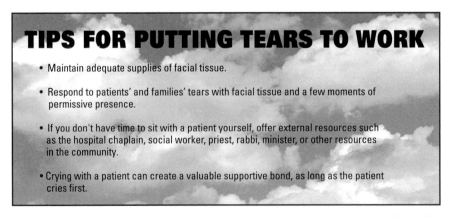

TIPS FOR PUTTING TEARS TO WORK

- Maintain adequate supplies of facial tissue.

- Respond to patients' and families' tears with facial tissue and a few moments of permissive presence.

- If you don't have time to sit with a patient yourself, offer external resources such as the hospital chaplain, social worker, priest, rabbi, minister, or other resources in the community.

- Crying with a patient can create a valuable supportive bond, as long as the patient cries first.

Tips for putting tears to work. (From Dugan, DO: Laughter and tears: Best medicine for stress. Nursing Forum 24:18, 1989. Reprinted with permission, Nursecom, Inc.)

imagine this scene. A beautiful little 4-year-old girl was severely brain injured in a car accident. She was in intensive care on a ventilator. The decision was made to take her off the ventilator, and her mother held her in a rocking chair and talked to her as the child died in her arms. It was a very sad night in the intensive care unit, not a dry eye in the house. Everyone on the unit was crying.

Sometimes you'll cry with patients and families; sometimes you'll cry in private. It's important to recognize, however, that when you cry, you're relieving your own emotional pain. Crying together with a patient or a family member can create a valuable and supportive bond. But you should avoid crying with a patient or family member unless that other person cries first. So what do you do when you feel like crying but need to remain in professional control? Try to bite your lip and pinch yourself, then excuse yourself from the room. Get behind closed doors to a safe and private place to let out your emotions. Talk about your feelings with a trusted colleague, who has undoubtedly had similar feelings and can help you sort through yours.

SUMMARY

Tears are a natural and effective way to release the tension that accompanies sadness, grief, anger, and fear. Family members may be grieving for the death or impending death of a loved one, or patients may be grieving for their own impending death and separation from loved ones. Patients and family members may be frustrated and angered to the point of tears, or they may be fearful or in pain. In each emotion, the sense of loss is the overriding feeling that leads to crying and tears. The list on page 206 summarizes how to put tears to work for your patient.[2]

Nursing a patient who feels a loss involves helping the person to feel "bad." It means helping the person experience painful emotions so that he can then experience the benefits of releasing tensions through tears. It also means supportively listening to the patient or family as they verbalize emotional pain. Therapeutic communication with a crying patient means that you avoid expressing disapproval or minimizing the cause for crying. Don't offer false hope or make promises you can't keep to convince the patient to stop crying. These behaviors may ease your own emotional discomfort, but they're not therapeutic.

COMMUNICATION EXERCISES

1 Write a one-page summary of a significant loss that you experienced. You may describe any loss, such as the loss of body image, loss of a loved one, or loss of a job. What were your feelings during the experience? What were your behaviors during the experience? How did you resolve your feelings of loss?

2 Break the class into small groups to discuss and summarize the feelings, behaviors, and ways of resolving feelings of loss identified in the first exercise. Have a designated leader tell the class the summary findings from each group. Identify differences in responses based on culture and gender. Identify healthy and unhealthy reactions to loss.

3 Use the following exercise to help come to grips with your own mortality. Suppose you are in a car accident and die tomorrow. List the relationships that would be lost. What should be done with your body? Would you want a funeral or memorial service? What would you want done with your property? List the uncompleted tasks you would leave behind. List activities that you should not put off any longer.

References

1. Glass, L: He Says, She Says: Closing the Communication Gap Between the Sexes. Berkley, New York, 1993.
2. Dugan, D: Laughter and tears: Best medicine for stress. Nursing Forum *24*:18, 1989.
3. Lindemann, E: Symptomatology and management of acute grief. American Journal of Psychiatry *101*:141, 1960.
4. Schulz, R: The Psychology of Death, Dying and Bereavement. Addison-Wesley, Reading, MA, 1978.
5. Kübler-Ross, E: To Live Until We Say Goodbye. Prentice-Hall: Englewood Cliffs, NJ, 1978.
6. Milliken, ME: Understanding Human Behavior, ed 5. Delmar: Albany, NY, 1993.
7. Erikson, EH: Childhood and Society, ed 2. Norton: New York, 1963.
8. Oates, WE: Your Particular Grief. The Westminster Press: Philadelphia, 1981.

Therapeutic Communication: The Foundation of Patient Education

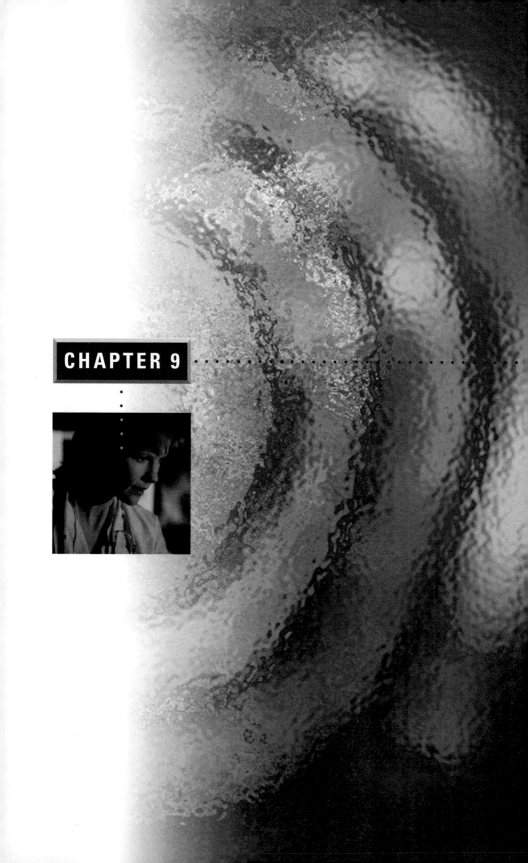

CHAPTER 9

Therapeutic Communication: The Foundation of Patient Education

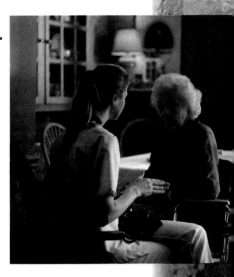

Chapter Objectives

AFTER READING THIS CHAPTER,
YOU WILL BE ABLE TO:

1. Describe the relationship between patient education and therapeutic communication.

2. Define learning and describe the cognitive, affective, and psychomotor aspects of learning.

3. Describe the basic principles of learning in adults and children.

4. Describe factors that inhibit and facilitate learning.

5. Identify basic content that all patients need to know for independent self-care.

6. Describe the basic assessment that must be done before making any attempt to teach the patient.

7. Identify the basic components of a teaching plan.

8. Identify the major teaching methods and relate them to the content to be taught.

9. Evaluate what the patient learned and the effectiveness of the teaching method.

10. Describe what to do when a patient decides not to follow the teachings and recommendations of health care providers.

N THIS CHAPTER, PRINCIPLES OF THERAPEUTIC COMMUNICATION ARE APPLIED to a very important nursing role: patient education. As you might expect, therapeutic communication is the foundation of patient educational processes.[1]

You'll need to integrate all of the communication assessment guidelines and communication techniques described in this book when educating patients. For example, the first step in teaching anything is to find out all you can about the person you're planning to teach. What is the patient's current reaction to the stress of illness? How is her self-esteem? Are any gender and cultural issues relevant to what you intend to teach? As you teach, you must constantly assess and analyze the patient and family to gauge what they've learned by how they communicate to you. And, of course, you'll use empathy, humor, and touch during patient education. Patients and family members will have confidence in what you teach them, and they'll retain more of what you teach them, when you effectively integrate therapeutic communication techniques into your teaching.

Basic Principles of Patient-Centered Learning

An important role for you as a nurse is to be a patient and family educator. However, many health care providers confuse teaching with telling. For example, in an outpatient setting, a health care provider may go into a room and tell the patient what he needs to do. The patient listens and nods as the person speaks. If the patient is lucky, he may be given a pamphlet to read. For example, the health care provider says, "As you know, your blood pressure is a little high. So is your cholesterol level. You need to lose 10 pounds by reducing your intake of fats and exercising at least three times a week. You'll also need to stop smoking. Here are pamphlets on diet, exercise, and smoking. You should also take your blood pressure every day and record it. Come back for a checkup in 3 months. Any questions?" The patient responds, "No."

Did the patient learn what the health care provider taught (told) him? Will the person go home and do what he was told? When (and if) the patient comes back in 3 months for a checkup, what are the chances he will have checked his blood pressure every day, lost 10 pounds, started exercising, and stopped smoking? The odds of accomplishing all these goals are very small indeed.

What's more, when the patient does come back for a checkup and his blood pressure and cholesterol are still high, he hasn't lost weight, and he hasn't stopped smoking, the patient may be labeled as "non-compliant" with the treatment plan. The problem is, however, that the health care provider told the patient what to do but neglected to explain how to do any of it. The fact is that exercising, dieting, measuring blood pressuring, and quitting smoking are massive behavioral changes that are easy to talk about but very difficult to do. These changes require alterations in comfortable, well-established lifestyle behaviors.

Instead of providing the kind of teaching described earlier, your patient education efforts must be firmly grounded in accepted principles of the teaching and learning process.[2,3] To teach means to impart knowledge so that learning can occur. Learning means that a change in cognitive knowledge, affective disposition, or physical behavioral capability has occurred that can't be accounted for by biological growth. Patient education implies that teachings are directed toward helping patients change their health-related cognitive knowledge, affective dispositions, and behavioral capabilities.

COGNITIVE KNOWLEDGE

The cognitive knowledge required to change behavior includes intellectual skills and the ability to comprehend and to apply knowledge to the lifestyle. Using the example given earlier, to obtain appropriate cognitive knowledge, the patient must learn *how* to change his diet, *how* to exercise, *how* to take a blood pressure, and *how* to quit smoking.

By telling a patient, "You must reduce your cholesterol, exercise, check your blood pressure, and stop smoking," as the health care provider in this example did, you assume that a patient has the cognitive knowledge he needs to accomplish those goals. You also assume that he's motivated enough to apply his knowledge to make numerous changes to his lifestyle. Clearly, these assumptions add up to a big mistake.

AFFECTIVE DISPOSITIONS

Affective dispositions include the attitudes, emotions, feelings, interests, and values of the patient. How motivated is the patient to make changes, and what support systems does he have to help him? In the previous example, the health care provider gave no consideration to how the patient felt about attempting to make significant changes in his life. Perhaps the patient really enjoys smoking, loves to eat at fast-food restaurants, and hates to exercise. Then what?

BEHAVIORAL CAPABILITIES

Behavioral capabilities are the psychomotor skills necessary for a change to occur. In the previous example, the patient was told to take his blood pressure every day. But the health care provider failed to determine whether the patient had the manual dexterity and the hearing acuity to take his own blood pressure. In fact, there's no way to validate those capabilities without having the patient give a return demonstration of the skill he'll be performing.

Clearly, learning is doomed to failure when a health care provider simply tells a patient what he needs to do without considering the cognitive, affective, and behavioral aspects of what he needs to learn. If the health care provider then wants to place blame on the patient for not following through on what he was told, she typically would label him noncompliant. However, you now can see why that term has received considerable criticism.

Besides its negative connotations, the term noncompliant assumes that health care professionals have the right to blame the patient when medical advice isn't implemented. It simply ignores the fact that the patient may not have the cognitive knowledge, affective dispositions, or behavioral skills that he needs—and that health care professionals should be taking the time to teach. What's more, remember that patients have the right to make their own decisions and to do whatever they believe is best for them, even when it goes against the medical advice they've received.

Adult Learning Principles

By implementing the following principles in your efforts to teach adult patients, you'll maximize your patients' success at learning. While you purposefully use these teaching strategies to facilitate participation, also make sure you're using appropriate therapeutic communication techniques, such as humor, touch, and empathy.

BUILD ON PREVIOUS EXPERIENCES

Adults learn by building on previous experiences. To teach an adult successfully, first find out his general experiences with illness and injury, and then address any misconceptions or fears he may have. It is especially relevant to find out about previous experiences that relate directly to the behaviors you're asking the patient to change. For instance, what does he know about diets, exercise, how to take a blood pressure reading, or how to stop smoking? What has he tried in the past? As with basic communication skills, go to where the patient is emotionally and cognitively, and build from there. Find ways to relate new learning to what he already knows and does.

FOCUS ON IMMEDIATE CONCERNS FIRST

Adults want to learn what they need to know *now*. They're interested in solving an immediate problem. So find out what the patient sees as an immediate problem. Always begin your teaching by finding the patient's immediate thoughts and needs. Adults must be involved in determining their own learning needs based on what they perceive to be the problem. Perhaps it's more of a problem to make the prescribed changes in lifestyle than to continue doing the same things they've been doing related to smoking, eating and exercising.

Blood pressure and cholesterol levels aren't visible and don't cause pain, so the patient may not view them as an immediate problem even though consequences will occur in the future. You must know whether the patient sees his health problem the same way you do or whether he sees it differently before you suggest which behaviors he should change or how he should go about changing them. Basic communication skills, such as active listening, clarifying, summarizing, and focusing are essential.

ADAPT TEACHING TO LIFESTYLE

To help your patient learn, you must tailor your teaching to make it relevant to the patient's present activities and responsibilities. You must take into consideration the patient's current lifestyle and make suggestions about how to modify it. If the patient eats out a lot, for example, help him learn to select low-fat foods from a menu.

If the patient doesn't cook and his wife is responsible for making the food, you're wasting time telling him how to modify recipes. His wife needs to be involved. Important considerations are the patient's age, occupation, educational level, self-concept, gender, and culture, all of which were discussed in various chapters throughout this book.

MAKE THE PATIENT AN ACTIVE PARTICIPANT

Adults prefer to be independent and in control of the learning process and outcome. The patient must determine his own learning needs. In addition, this means the patient must actively participate. Teaching methods must be selected to facilitate active participation. Learning is faster and retention is better with the active involvement of the learner.

You should plan to have open discussions (not lectures), which are effective teaching strategies for cognitive and affective content. Encourage the patient to ask questions to clarify material. You should ask questions, too, to validate what the patient learned.

Lecturing may be appropriate in classroom situations with large groups of patients, but it's not appropriate for individual patient teaching sessions. Lecturing is not appropriate because it allows no interaction. Also, it puts the teacher in charge while placing the learner in a dependent and passive role.[4] To teach psychomotor skills, you'll need to use demonstrations. The patient becomes actively involved in giving return demonstrations to validate learning.

Learning in Children

All that has been said about teaching adults applies to teaching children. Of course, you must always include the parents and obtain their cooperation in your teaching. Most important, you'll need to take the child's stage of cognitive development into consideration, as outlined here.[5,6]

From birth to age 2 years, a child learns to differentiate herself from her surroundings. She learns that her actions have effects on people and objects. Your teaching should be aimed at the parents while making the child feel as secure and comfortable as possible.

From ages 2 to 7, a child is in the stage of preoperational development. She takes everything literally and cannot generalize. She can manipulate equipment and be shown how to use equipment. Use simple terms and be matter of fact. Have the child practice on a doll. Encourage her to express her fears, and don't make false promises. If it will hurt, don't say that it won't.

From ages 7 to 12, children develop concrete operational thoughts. By age 12, a child can understand cause-and-effect relationships and has developed logical reasoning abilities. To teach her, use simple drawings and the correct medical equipment for explanations. You can relate stories of other children's problems, and she'll probably understand your analogy.

From ages 12 to 18, children have well developed cognitive abilities. At this stage, you can provide more technical information if the patient wants to know more about what's going on. Children of these ages are also working to establish independence, and just like adults, they may resent being told what to do by health care providers. Give a teenager a chance to discuss her feelings without her parents being present, and reassure her that you will keep her thoughts and feelings confidential.

Steps to Facilitate Learning

There are a number of things you can do to facilitate learning and optimize your effectiveness as a teacher.

ASSESS THE LEARNER

Always start by assessing the learner. As you go into a room with teaching as your goal, always find out first what the patient's immediate thoughts and needs are. These immediate thoughts and needs may not be related to teaching or learning at all. Nevertheless, you'll need to address them first. Afterward, the patient will be much more willing and able to learn. For instance, suppose you enter a patient's room and find out that she's in pain. You'll need to do something to control the pain before you can start to teach. A person in pain can't concentrate.

Once you have assessed the patient's general concerns, you can begin teaching by determining how well she understands the health care problem you'll be discussing. Does the patient know what's wrong with her and what caused it? Does she know what to do to prevent it from happening again? Does she know the signs and symptoms of the problem should it recur? What concerns this patient the most? To help keep your teaching accurately focused, you'll want to ask the patient open-ended questions to address all these areas of learning. Allow the patient to express herself freely; doing so may give you an idea about where to start teaching. Try to get a sense of the patient's viewpoint and priorities, and then you can personalize your teachings.[3]

This idea relates well with the basic therapeutic communication principle of building rapport. Learning is more likely to occur if the patient trusts you, respects you, and believes that you're trying to help her with a problem.

READINESS TO LEARN

You'll also need to determine whether the patient is ready, willing, and able to learn. If the person is in pain, tired, hungry, anxious, fearful, in denial, or distracted, you're wasting time by trying to teach; learning will not take place. You will need to postpone teaching, or perhaps redirect what needs to be learned to a family member who will be assisting in the care of the patient.

Say, for example, that a patient came up from the cardiac catheterization lab around noon. The patient was tired after being in the lab for about 3 hours for testing. The patient was also hungry because he wasn't allowed to eat before the test and lunch hadn't yet been delivered. The patient also was uncomfortable because he had to stay in bed and lie still with a pressure dressing and sand bag on the leg that had been catheterized. At that point, the dietitian walked in, pulled up a chair, and started teaching him about a low-fat, low-salt cardiac diet.

How much do you imagine the patient learned about the diet? Probably nothing. If the health care provider had assessed the patient first and applied basic principles of teaching, he would have known to leave this patient alone until he had eaten and rested. The patient was polite and said nothing, although some patients might have said, "I'm tired, hungry, and uncomfortable. Can you come back later when I can actually hear what you're trying to tell me?" Even if the patient doesn't speak up, however, you'll have clues to his learning readiness. If at any point during a teaching session, a patient's eyes glaze over and he looks out into space, you've lost him.

FIRST THINGS FIRST

Remember always to let the patient's learning needs direct your teaching. Once you have identified the patient's most urgent concerns, address these areas first, even though you've planned a sequence to your teaching and knew what you wanted to cover first, second, and third. Patients will be self-motivated to address their most urgent concerns, and they'll tune in closely to what you are trying to teach in those areas.

BE REALISTIC

Throughout your teaching, be realistic and stick to the basics. Tailor the information you present so the goals are attainable by the patient you're teaching. Remember that the average adult can remember only five to seven things at a time, so keep your teachings short, simple, and specific. The more information you present, the more the patient will forget. Less information is really more, because the information will be better retained. Never try to present everything in one teaching session. Teaching small amounts of information over time is much more effective.[7]

For example, a realistic goal may be to teach a patient about a medication he needs for hypertension. You can include the name of the medication, how it helps, when to take it, adverse effects it might cause, and what to do if any of those effects arise. Separate nice-to-know information from essential information, and concentrate on the essentials. In this drug example, you'd skip how the drug is metabolized in the body, and you wouldn't need to discuss every rare adverse effect experienced by everyone taking the drug.

In addition, use simple everyday language, avoiding medical terminology whenever possible. There is a big difference between saying "Let's talk about how to increase the oxygenation of your blood," and saying "Let's talk about what to do when you feel short of breath." You've said the same thing, but the nonmedical description will be much more likely to get the patient's attention and understanding.

Also, be very clear and specific with directions. If your discharge instruction sheet says that a dressing should be removed in a few days, the patient won't know who's supposed to remove it or how many days you consider to be "a few."

TIMING IS EVERYTHING

Take advantage of each teachable moment.[3] You can make the most of your time and the patient's time by incorporating teaching into your ongoing patient care. Each time you are with a patient, you can teach and validate what has been taught before. As you change a dressing, you can discuss wound care or signs and symptoms of infection. As you administer medications, you can ask what each is for. As you walk with a patient, you can discuss home exercises. Take action at every teachable moment. In addition, keep the time between learning the information and applying the information as short as possible to help the patient retain the information.

You can also make the most of your time by involving the patient's family in the teaching. Have family members present whenever possible. They can reinforce instructions. Also, what one person doesn't remember, the other person may remember. They may also encourage the patient to do what is needed and support her in making behavioral changes. For example, say a patient has just returned from surgery and the family is in the room. Although the patient is still groggy from anesthesia and pain medications, you ask her to do routine postoperative breathing and leg exercises, and you explain to the family what you are doing and why. You also ask them to remind the patient to do these exercises every hour while awake to prevent postoperative complications.

REINFORCE ALL LEARNING

It's crucial that you remember to give positive reinforcement each time the patient takes a step toward making a change—even a small step. Reward the patient by praising her progress with a few words, a smile, or a pat on the back.

Continue to review the material you're taught, recognizing that change takes time and practice. In a hospital setting, you can review teaching material over the course of each shift. In a home setting or clinic, you'll need to review each time you have an appointment with the patient. Document your teaching and the patient's progress. Also communicate these ideas to other health care professionals who will care for the patient. Share information about what the patient has learned and what still requires more teaching and reinforcement. Also, let your colleagues know which teaching methods were and were not effective for this patient.

You may also want to refer a patient to a support group for ongoing help with making needed changes, reinforcing behaviors, and maintaining behavior changes. For the patient with high cholesterol and a need for dietary modification, you might make a referral to an organization such as Weight Watchers rather than simply telling the patient to go on a low-fat diet and start exercising.

SOLICIT FEEDBACK

You must verify all messages you send by paying careful attention to feedback. In the case of patient education, the feedback is in the form of evaluating what the patient has learned. This is an extremely important part of patient education. Unfortunately, in many patient care situations, evaluation is rarely done. But how can you know if your patient learned something unless you solicit feedback from him? Just because you go over information with someone, you can't assume that he knows what you mean or knows how to do what you asked.

How do you evaluate what a patient knows? In most cases, giving a written test isn't appropriate. Start an evaluation by asking if the patient has any questions after you present information or finish your discussion. After you address these questions, you need to ask some additional questions to confirm the patient's understanding. Ask her to restate information, for example, "Let's review a little bit so I know that I clearly explained the signs of bladder infection to you. Can you tell me what signs you should watch for that might mean you have an infection in your bladder?"

Another excellent way to find out what a patient has learned is by giving her a brief scenario that relates to her life and then asking how she'd handle it. For example, "I want to be sure I'm explaining this clearly to you, so let me give you this example. Say you feel some pressure and burning when you urinate. What does that mean, and what should you do about it?" You can evaluate both cognitive and affective forms of learning with oral questions.

Return demonstrations are the only way to evaluate performance of a psychomotor skill.[8] Suppose the patient with recurrent bladder infections from the previous example needs also to be taught self-catheterization. The only way you'll know for sure that she can do the procedure is by watching her catheterize herself using the exact same equipment she'll be using when performing the procedure alone. Even if the patient can tell you the steps in the procedure and even if she can do the procedure on a mannequin, you still need to validate that she really has the psychomotor skills to perform the procedure on herself. For that, you need a return demonstration.

Factors That Inhibit Learning

Nurses must keep in mind several factors that can inhibit learning. When these factors are present, they must be under control before learning can occur.

EMOTIONS

Are you remembering always to deal with emotions first when working with a patient? Always evaluate her emotional state first before teaching or doing *anything* else. Emotions are a prime consideration as you communicate, either when teaching or attempting any other form of communication.

A basic teaching rule is that as anxiety increases, learning decreases. A little bit of anxiety may be motivating, but too much anxiety prevents the patient from focusing. Her anxiety must be reduced. Sometimes, therapeutic touch or humor can be very useful in reducing anxiety, as described in Chapters 6 and 7.

You must also be aware of the patient's state of depression and grief related to illness and the temporary or permanent loss of abilities. Sometimes you can instill hope by relating similar cases with positive outcomes or relating progress made in treating a particular disease. If the patient thinks that there's no way she can handle a situation and she feels overwhelmed, she won't be capable of learning at that time. For example, consider a patient who is in her second day after unexpected cardiac surgery. She's lying in bed thinking how difficult it is to get from the bed to the chair with chest tubes and oxygen going. Just then, the rehabilitation nurse comes in to review the walking exercises the patient should be doing after discharge. Before wasting time on these instructions, which the patient won't hear, the nurse should assess the patient's perception of exercise at that time and build up her confidence before attempting to teach.

DEFENSE MECHANISMS

A patient who is in denial about an illness or rationalizing about why he can't do something will need to get beyond that point before he'll be able to make a change in behavior. For example, say you're teaching a class on smoking cessation to patients with high blood pressure. You have explained risk factors and statistics, and the patients can repeat them to you. They have cognitive knowledge. Next, one of the patients tells you that his grandfather smoked and lived to be 90 years old. The patient then reminds you that lots of people with high blood pressure don't smoke. This patient is using defense mechanisms. Don't argue with him, and don't repeat your lecture; the patient already heard it. At this point, for this patient, your teaching should be aimed at increasing his awareness of the condition. You may be able to teach him to monitor his blood pressure and record it. Then see if you can get the patient to cut down a little on cigarettes and see what happens to his blood pressure.

PHYSIOLOGICAL PROBLEMS

A patient's physiological state can interfere with learning also. When someone is too tired, hungry, in pain, nauseated, or vomiting, you'll need to postpone your lesson until the physiological problem has been resolved. If the patient is blind, has impaired hearing, or doesn't have the strength or coordination to do what is required, you must gear your teaching toward a family member who will care for the patient. As an option, you could also make referrals to appropriate outside agencies to assist with whatever needs to be done.

CULTURAL BARRIERS

Often, patients and family members have values that differ from yours and those of other health care providers. For example, say you explain to an Amish man that he needs an electric implanted defibrillator to control his heart arrhythmia or he'll die. But Amish people don't have electricity in their homes, and they still drive horses and buggies because they believe modern conveniences, such as electricity and cars, are the work of the devil. This patient may well choose to die rather than have an electrical device implanted in his body.

Sometimes you'll need to accept a patient's beliefs and avoid trying to impose the values of the medical community on him. In this example, you must not castigate the patient for his decision not to accept the electrical device. Instead, his physician will most likely prescribe medications to control the arrhythmia at least partly. Perhaps this isn't the best solution to solve the problem from a medical perspective. But certainly, from the patient's perspective, it is the best solution.

Understanding cultural differences will help you adapt what and how you teach to specific practices and beliefs. For example, a low-fat diet and menus can be tailored to satisfy the requirements of a particular culture. Italian spaghetti, German potato salad, French onion soup, Mexican tacos, or any other specific foods can be modified for a low-fat diet. The teaching will be better received because you have taken into consideration the lifestyle of an individual and suggested modifications that are realistic and acceptable.

Basic Content: What all Patients and Families Should Know

Most student nurses wonder where to begin teaching about a particular health issue and how to determine when they've covered all the essential information. There's a basic set of information that all patients and families should know about a particular health issue. No matter what kind of health care setting you work in, your patient teaching will be directed at key areas. The goal is to make patients as independent as possible in providing their own self-care in all settings. You can use the acronym METHOD[9] to remember what patients and family members need to know to provide self-care:

- M is for medications
- E is for environment
- T is for treatments
- H is for health knowledge about the disease
- O is for outpatient referrals
- D is for diet.

The following are very basic guidelines for what you should teach patients and families to ensure appropriate self-care. In addition to using these basic guidelines, also make sure that you read any patient education literature before giving that literature to your patients. Reading this literature can help you remember which details to include when teaching about a particular problem.

MEDICATIONS

All patients and family caretakers need to know the names and dosages of each drug that the patient must take. They must know what the drugs are for, what time the drugs should be taken, and how the drugs should be taken. They must also know the common side effects of each drug and which side effects should prompt a call to the doctor or nurse practitioner.

Write down the name of each medication, and include all the information needed in words that the patient can understand. Many times, standardized written patient education drug guidelines are available to be used as an adjunct to teaching. Any special instructions can be written on these standardized medication guidelines.

For example, a patient prone to congestive heart failure will take Lanoxin (brand name), also called digoxin (generic name), 0.125 mg, one time daily to help his heart beat strongly. You'll need to teach him to take his pulse before taking the drug, and to call his doctor before taking the drug if his pulse is below 60 beats per minute. You'll also need to explain the drug's most common side effects, including fatigue, nausea, vomiting, diarrhea, and blurred or yellow vision. Teach him to call his doctor immediately if any of these problems develop. Urge the patient to take the drug exactly as prescribed to help it be effective. Warn the patient never to double up on the drug if he forgets a dose because too much of the drug in the system at one time can cause pronounced side effects. Tell him that the doctor will want to monitor the level of the drug in his blood, and that the patient will need to have his blood drawn and checked in 2 weeks.

To reinforce your teaching about medications, each time you give any pill, check the patient's knowledge by asking, "What is this for?" Also ask, "When do you take this at home?" and, "Let's take your pulse together and compare what we get." It only takes a few minutes if you plan to integrate education into whatever you're doing.

ENVIRONMENT

Often a patient's environment will need to be modified to accommodate his health problem. For example, the patient's home environment might need to be modified by obtaining a portable toilet if the patient with heart problems can't go up and down the stairs. A portable phone may need to be obtained so it can be near the patient as he lies down to rest.

Take time to consider the modifications your patient's environment will need to accommodate him. Also, always check to be sure that the patient has the means to pay for whatever is needed. You can spend all the time in the world teaching the patient how and what to do, but your teaching will be useless if you fail to find out whether the patient can afford to follow your teaching. Many types of equipment and medications are very expensive, and some patients may not have equipment or prescription benefits in their health care plans. An example is a man who had high blood pressure who took his pills only when he checked his blood pressure and it was high. If it wasn't high, he didn't take his pills because they were expensive.

He continued this behavior even after the nurse and doctor at the clinic carefully explained the nature of hypertension and why it was so important to take his antihypertensive medication regularly. When he returned to the clinic 2 months later, the patient dejectedly asked if there was anything else he could take for his blood pressure because he just couldn't afford the current prescription. The lesson to be learned here is this: Don't assume that patients can afford to follow your teachings. One of the primary things you may to need to teach is how to get financial assistance to pay for the needed care. If you are not familiar with types of financial aid, then make a referral to another person in your own agency or outside agency, such as a government office of human services or the social service department where you work.

Family members in the patient's environment must be prepared to adapt as well, so they don't expect too much or too little of the patient's functional abilities. Include the family in whatever teaching you give the patient whenever possible. Always make explanations to the patient and any interested family members. When family members are in the same room as you and the patient, as they often are in hospital or home settings, include them and make them feel welcome. Family physical and emotional support is crucial to successful outcomes. However, remember that not everyone has a supportive family, and you can't assume that the patients do. Assess family reactions and responses just as you assess the patient's.

TREATMENTS

Treatments include any procedures that the patient must learn to do. For example, the patient and family may need to learn to change a dressing, perform self-injections, perform self-catheterization, administer oxygen, and so on. Teaching involves demonstration of how to do the procedure and always includes a return demonstration by the patient. Also included in the teaching is how to obtain supplies needed for the procedure.

Remember that affective behaviors are very important to performing self-procedures. What if the patient just can't stand to look at the wound under the dressing he's supposed to change? It's time to call on family members to see if they can help. If not, you'll need to make a referral.

HEALTH KNOWLEDGE

The patient needs cognitive knowledge of his health problem, including important details of the disease and the signs and symptoms that require immediate attention. For example, a patient with congestive heart failure needs to know that his heart isn't pumping as efficiently as it used to. To keep track of this condition, he should monitor his weight. In addition, he needs to look for swelling in his ankles, watch for shortness of breath, and feelings of chest tightness or pain. These are all signs that the heart isn't pumping efficiently. If he gains more than 2 pounds in a day, or if he experiences any of the other signs and symptoms listed, he should call his doctor right away.

In addition, he'll need to know about any activity limitations created by the condition. Telling a patient, "Go home and take it easy," is a classic educational blunder on the part of health care providers. Exactly what does "Take it easy" mean? Another activity guide that is vague yet often told to patients is, "You can only do light activities." Again, what does that mean? You need to be specific. Give some examples. Light activities means peeling potatoes while sitting down, watching TV, ironing while sitting down, reading the newspaper, and so on. For the first 3 days at home, the patient shouldn't stand up for more than 20 minutes without taking a brief 5-minute break to sit down. He shouldn't lift groceries, children, or anything else of similar weight. He should minimize trips up and down stairs to once in the morning and once at night.

Exercise guidelines are very important. Directions include walking around in the home. Teach him to walk up and down the driveway three times each day—once in the morning, once at noon, and once at night. Usually after major surgery or childbirth, a patient can resume (or start) a regular exercise schedule in about 6 weeks. Healing takes that long to occur. Patients must start out gradually and build up to 30 minutes three times weekly with warm-up and cool-down activities. The patient should start with 5 minutes of walking and build up gradually to 30 minutes.

Sexual activities must also be discussed. For example, with prostate surgery, rectovaginal surgery, or childbirth, it may take 5 to 6 weeks before it's safe to resume sexual activity to allow healing and avoid infection. "No douching, no tampons, no sex" for that period of time are the typical instructions after gynecological surgery or childbirth to prevent infections. A general rule of thumb for heart patients is that if they can tolerate climbing two flights of stairs, they can have sexual activity with their usual partner. Sexual activities, however, may be hindered by complications such as emotional barriers or impotence caused by medications or surgery.

Driving is a very important activity to be discussed. For example, patients must not drive while taking pain medications that act as central nervous system depressants. Other drugs may require a period of adjustment before the patient can safely drive or operate dangerous equipment (such as an electric saw).

When the patient can return to work is also very important. Return to work varies with the type of exertion required on the job. An office worker can return sooner that a laborer in most cases. In some situations, patients may need some form of occupational therapy or job retraining, and you'll need to make appropriate referrals.

OUTPATIENT REFERRALS

The patient and family must be informed about when they should be seen again by a health care provider. When is the next clinic or doctor's office appointment? Will the patient need the services of other agencies, such as home health care for intravenous therapy, hospice, or other private agencies? In addition, the patient may need referrals to community agencies for supportive services, such as the American Heart Association, American Cancer Society, ostomy organizations, mastectomy organizations, and so on. When making referrals or telling patients about an appointment at a certain date and time, don't assume that they own a car or know how to drive. They may need a family member's help or a community transportation service.

DIET

Patients and families need to be aware of special diets to be followed. Dietary restrictions and sample menus should be provided, and they should receive counseling from a dietitian as necessary. You should encourage them to eat foods that promote healing and health in general. For example, patients should be encouraged to select and prepare foods that have reduced fat, such as baked meats instead of fried meats. Protein is essential for wound healing. In general, patients should be encouraged to use salt in moderation. Too much salt causes fluid retention and contributes to hypertension.

In addition, foods that are high in fiber and rich in vitamins and minerals, such as fruits and vegetables, should be encouraged to prevent constipation and promote healing. Almost everyone should drink eight glasses of water a day unless there's a medical reason for fluid restriction. A basic healthy diet that could be used as a general guide is shown on page 229. The general guidelines need to be modified and adapted depending on the foods the patient likes to eat and any restrictions imposed by the disease.

Patient Assessment: The Critical First Step

Once you've got the basic principles of teaching and learning firmly rooted in your mind, begin to teach by assessing the patient. Each and every one of the questions you ask a patient needs to be done using therapeutic techniques. Some of the information may be obtained from patient records, but the rest can come only from the patient. Therapeutic communication skills are essential. Although some of these assessment areas were described earlier in the chapter, below is a summary of what you need to know about the patient and the situation before developing a teaching plan.

AGE

Age is important in assessing the patient's developmental tasks and cognitive level of development. What are the typical developmental tasks and what is the typical cognitive level of development at this age? Your general approach to teaching will be related to the age of the patient. An open-ended question to assess what the problem means to the patient from a developmental perspective is "How do you think this will change your life?"

CURRENT UNDERSTANDING OF THE HEALTH PROBLEM

Don't assume that a patient knows anything about the problem and how to handle it without asking questions. Ask, "What has the doctor been telling you about the problem?" to assess the patient's basic understanding about the problem. Ask, "What has the doctor been telling you about options available to treat the condition?" Ask, "Do you know what caused the problem?" Also, "What concerns you the most right now?"

HEALTHY DIET TIPS

Meats
- Increase chicken (skinless and not fried), fish, turkey, and tuna.
- Decrease red meat, eggs, and processed meat.

Dairy
- Increase low-fat milk (skim, .5%, 1%, or 2%), low-fat yogurt, and low-fat cottage cheese.
- Decrease cheese and ice cream.

Grains and Cereals
- Increase bran fiber, whole wheat bread, bran cereals, rice, and potatoes.
- Decrease white breads and buns.

Fruits and Vegetables
- Increase fresh or frozen fruit and vegetables, salads, and fruit juices.
- Decrease canned vegetables and fruits packed in syrup.

Fluids
- Drink 8 glasses of water each day.
- Limit caffeine to one or two servings per day of cola, coffee, or tea.

Other
- Decrease salt by avoiding table salt, processed foods, canned foods and soups, pizza, pickles, and lunchmeat.
- Decrease fat and cholesterol by limiting red meats, butter (margarine only), high-fat dairy products (such as cheese and ice cream), eggs, peanut butter, and nuts. Skin all poultry.
- Avoid the following except on special occasions: candy, cake, pie, cookies, ice cream, and chips and dip. Even on special occasions, minimize consumption of these foods.

Healthy diet tips.

EFFECTS OF GENDER AND CULTURE

What is the patient's cultural background? What practices may be related to what you're trying to teach? As you teach about diet, have you considered food preferences based on culture and made modifications to the standard teaching aids to fit this patient's background? In some cultures, women are the primary caretakers and will need to be involved in all teachings as they attempt to take responsibility for their spouse's welfare.

ECONOMICS

You must know how much the drugs, dressings, and other needed supplies will cost the patient, whether the patient's health plan will cover them, and whether the patient can afford what's left over after the insurance is finished. In other words, how much will the patient be expected to pay out of pocket? The reality for many patients is that they can't afford what nurses teach them to do. If that's the case, you'll need to separate the essentials from the alternatives. For example, perhaps a generic drug can be substituted for the more expensive brand name drug.

SUPPORT SYSTEMS

What family and friends are available to the patient? Are they supportive of the patient emotionally? Do they agree that the treatments are appropriate? Ask, "How has the illness effected your family?" Consider, for example, an 88-year-old grandmother living in her own home. She's scheduled to have physical therapy to improve the range of motion in her joints. She can't drive herself to the appointment, so a family member will have to do it. It's important for you to find out whether the patient's family agrees that physical therapy is important, or whether they think it's a waste of time. If they think it is a waste, they'll be reluctant to take time to drive her to the appointment. They may even discourage her from going. What if they agree that physical therapy is important but they don't have the time to take her to the appointments three times a week? The solution may be to enroll in a physical therapy center that has a bus service for patients.

READINESS AND MOTIVATION

Is the patient ready and motivated to learn at this time? Has she accepted her situation and decided that she wants to improve it? Is she physically able to learn at this time without pain, nausea, or fatigue? If she's anxious or fearful, find out about what. Not every patient has the same fears and anxieties, so an open-ended statement, such as, "Tell me more about your fear" is appropriate. For example, the patient may say, "I'm afraid to be put to sleep for surgery." When you ask a more detailed question, you then find out that she had a friend who developed malignant hyperthermia and died while under anesthesia. Or you may find out that the patient fears waking up too soon during the surgery. Don't assume that you know what the patient fears. Ask the patient to tell you. If the patient is a little anxious, try calming her with reassurance and some light humor so she'll be better able to relax and retain your teaching.

LEARNING STYLE AND READING LEVEL

Learning styles are how people learn best. Questions to ask patients to try to figure out how they will learn best are as follows:

- "Do you learn best by having someone go over everything point by point?"
- "Would you prefer to watch a video, listen to an audiotape, use a computerized learning program, or read by yourself first and then ask questions?"
- "Can you hear and see me okay?" With a patient who is sight impaired, large-size print materials or audio tapes might work best. With a patient who can't hear, printed materials and videotapes with subtitles can be useful. Also with patients who have hearing impairments, speak slowly and distinctly, and ask them to repeat back to you frequently to make sure they've heard what you said. Sometimes it may look like a person is hearing you, but if you ask them to repeat it, they can't.

A prime consideration is the patient's reading level. Many patients who are illiterate may be too embarrassed to admit it. One of five adults reads at a fifth-grade level or lower. A tactful way to evaluate reading is to ask, "Do you like to read?" If the answer is no, you'll need to find another way to present the information without embarrassing the person. If he wears glasses, does he have them with him? Most people beyond age 40 have special glasses for reading. Although there is written patient teaching literature readily available on almost any topic, you must evaluate whether the patient can read it first, and then whether he can comprehend and apply it to his personal situation.

Major Components of a Teaching Plan

Now that you know basically what you are supposed to be teaching and how to do a basic assessment, you need to develop a plan with specific goals and objectives, and with teaching methods for each goal and objective. The plan has to be specific and individualized to what you assessed about the patient.

ASSESSMENT

Let's say you've done the assessment described earlier and found that the patient has a knowledge deficit about his newly diagnosed diabetes and the need to take insulin. He first wants to learn about insulin and how to give his own injections. This scenario is comically depicted in the cartoon on page 233. He is 55 years old, has a college degree, has been an investment broker for the past 25 years, and wants to get back to his work as soon as possible. He is motivated to learn, he likes to read, and his family is supportive. His wife wants to attend nutrition classes to learn the new diet and how to modify the way she currently cooks. The patient's insurance plan covers prescription medications and the supplies needed for injecting insulin.

GOALS AND OBJECTIVES

Based on this assessment, your general goal will be to have the patient independently administer insulin. You must write specific objectives to address cognitive, affective, and psychomotor learning behaviors that the patient must attain to successfully meet the goal. These are examples of learning objectives that are specifically designed to meet the needs of the patient. Cognitive learning objectives specify that the patient do the following:

- Describes what the drug insulin is for
- Describes the adverse effects of too much or too little insulin
- States what to do if side effects occur.

Affective learning objectives specify that the patient should do the following:

- Listens to instructions on how to give an injection
- States that an injection is necessary and why it is necessary
- Shows no signs of anxiety and appears relaxed.

Psychomotor learning objectives specify the patient do the following:

- Assembles supplies needed to self-administer insulin
- Draws into the syringe the correct dosage of the drug without contaminating the equipment
- Injects insulin without contaminating the needle.

Note that the above-mentioned objectives are clearly measurable. This means that by reading the objective, you can identify a specific thing the patient will do or say to let you know when he has accomplished the objective.

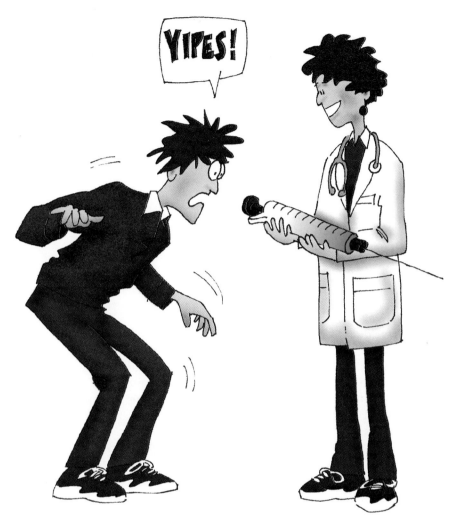

Even a mature person with substantial responsibilities may have much to learn about an illness and its treatment.

TEACHING STRATEGIES

Next, you must plan the teaching strategies that will best meet the objectives. The strategies discussed in the following sections are grouped according to whether learning objectives are cognitive, affective, or psychomotor.

Cognitive Objectives

Cognitive knowledge is usually taught using printed and audiovisual materials. These strategies include books, pamphlets, films, programmed instruction, and computer learning. The learner can proceed at his own pace, and you don't need to be present during learning. You act as a resource person and answer the patient's questions or concerns. This is potentially ineffective if the reading level of the material is too high.

Cognitive knowledge can also be learned when you give explanations and descriptions. You control the content and the pace of the instruction, and the learner is passive and will retain less information than when an active participant in the learning process.

In addition, cognitive knowledge may be gained by encouraging the patient to ask questions. The patient must feel comfortable asking questions and not be concerned that he'll embarrass himself by asking a "dumb" question or embarrass you by asking a "private" question. You'll need to confirm that each question has been answered by asking the learner, "Does that answer your question?"

Affective and Cognitive Objectives

Affective and cognitive knowledge can be gained from one-to-one discussion that permits the introduction of sensitive issues and encourages participation by the learner. You can provide immediate reinforcement and as much repetition as needed until the patient learns the objectives of the lesson. Group discussions may also be useful for affective and cognitive knowledge when the group members are supportive of each other, share their ideas and concerns, and problem-solve together.

Role playing may also be a useful tool for affective and cognitive knowledge because it permits the expression of attitudes, values, and emotions, and it allows active involvement by the learner. In addition, affective and cognitive behaviors may be learned by the strategy of discovery. Using discovery, you guide the patient through problem-solving situations. The patient is an active participant, and retention of information is high.

Psychomotor Objectives

Psychomotor skills are initially taught by demonstrations accompanied by explanations. However, demonstration alone isn't effective for learning a psychomotor skill because the learner is passive. Therefore, demonstrations must be accompanied by the teaching strategy of guided practice. The patient must have "hands-on" experience, with repetition and immediate feedback from you.

In addition, other patients who have previously mastered the techniques may serve as models for psychomotor behavioral skills. They set an example for patients who are newly diagnosed and in the process of learning new behaviors. The patient must be able to identify with the model for the strategy to be effective.

To individualize the teaching of the diabetic patient in the example used earlier, you would select pamphlets on insulin and insulin administration. Pamphlets and reading materials are often effective strategies to accomplish the cognitive objectives of describing insulin, learning the side effects of too much or too little insulin, and learning what to do if side effects occur. Then you could have a time for questions and answers to follow up on the patient's grasp of the reading materials. A videotape of a patient drawing up and self-administering insulin in the home setting can serve as a model of the expected behavior. Then you can demonstrate drawing up and giving insulin, and the patient can try it as many times as necessary to master the psychomotor skill. One-to-one discussion can be used for the affective objectives of the willingness to listen, the acceptance of the need for the injections, and the presence of anxiety.

IMPLEMENTATION OF TEACHING

After developing the plan, it's now time for patient-nurse interaction. Make sure to choose a good time for the interaction. A good time might be after breakfast, after the patient has slept well, when the patient has no discomforts and is ready to learn. This environment is optimal.

Order the learning activities by starting with the basics. Give the patient the pamphlets, and tell the patient that you'll return in an hour to talk about his questions. When you return, answer his questions and have a one-to-one discussion regarding affective behaviors. Next, take the patient to a small classroom where the movie and equipment are prepared ahead of time. Play the movie, give a live demonstration, and follow this up with practice by the patient on a mannequin. Last, have the patient self-inject sterile water.

EVALUATION AND DOCUMENTATION OF LEARNING AND TEACHING

The last step in the teaching and learning process is to evaluate whether learning occurred and the teaching methods were effective, and to document what was done. In order to evaluate, ask yourself, "Did the patient learn about insulin and how to give the injection?" More specifically, ask yourself, "Did the patient master each of the objectives?"

How do we know if the objectives are mastered or not? You must specifically evaluate each objective. Typically, cognitive objectives can be evaluated by giving the patient a test, oral or written. You can also have the patient keep a diary or records for self-monitoring.

Affective behaviors can be inferred from *how* the client responds to questions and *how* he speaks about relevant topics. In addition, you can observe behaviors that express feelings and values.

Psychomotor behaviors can be measured by only direct observation. The patient may be able to describe each step in the procedure, but this ability simply demonstrates cognitive knowledge, not psychomotor competence. Therefore, you must observe the patient directly performing the activity.

To continue with the example of the diabetic patient, you will evaluate cognitive knowledge by asking oral questions and giving the patient examples of situations for which he'd describe his response. For example, "You're driving in your car about 11 am after giving yourself insulin at 8 am. You become light-headed, you start sweating, and you feel shaky. What do you think is wrong and what should you do?" Next you evaluate the patient's psychomotor abilities by telling him to pretend that you're not there and to do everything needed to draw up and administer the injection just like he'll be doing at home. In addition, you simultaneously evaluate his affective behaviors by noting how he responds to your questions and how his facial expressions change as he gives himself an injection.

Last is the evaluation of your teaching methods. Was the timing of your teaching appropriate? Were your strategies effective? Was the amount of information appropriate? You can ask your patient for insight either orally or in writing. By evaluating oral or written responses, you can tell whether your objectives were met or not. Other characteristics of effective teaching include the ability to hold the patient's interest and the ability to make the patient a partner—an active participant—in the teaching and learning process. Good teachers are also optimistic, positive, nonthreatening, and supportive of a positive self-concept in learners. They help patients believe that they can accomplish all objectives. Last, a good teacher typically uses several methods of teaching that are appropriate for the objectives and the learning style of the patient.

When a Patient Decides not To Change a Behavior

You've done everything to convince a patient to change a behavior to become healthier. You've tried every teaching method to present cognitive knowledge. The patient just doesn't want to stop smoking. Now what? You can do no more. Don't keep repeating yourself over and over. Don't get into an argument. You must agree that you disagree, and that ultimately, patients have the right to their own opinions and decisions. You can't force anyone to do something they don't want to do. You gave it your best shot. Not every patient wants to learn or change an established pattern of behavior. Sometimes the best you can do in this situation is assess readiness, document your findings, and communicate with other health care providers.

For example, say the patient has lung cancer and doesn't want to stop smoking but will be seeing a visiting nurse three times a week at his home. You can let the visiting nurse know the problem, what you've taught the patient, and the patient's response. Then let this nurse carry on, watching for the teachable moment when the patient is motivated to change the smoking behavior.

SUMMARY

Patient education is a very important nursing responsibility that involves the application of the principles of therapeutic communication. Therapeutic communication must be used throughout the teaching and learning process. In this chapter, basic principles of teaching and learning are described. To perform this important task properly, you must develop knowledge of how to perform a learning assessment, develop a teaching plan, administer the teaching, and evaluate learning and teaching strategies. You also must realize that not everyone is willing (or able) to change their behaviors. Although a patient has the cognitive knowledge needed for change, he may still decide against it. Ultimately, it's the patient's right to decide whether or not to make a lifestyle change.

COMMUNICATION EXERCISES

1 The following patients are newly diagnosed with diabetes and require insulin to control the disease. Each has a particular learning need. In Case 1, the patient is legally blind. In Case 2, the patient has been up all night because of a very noisy roommate and feels very tired. In Case 3, the patient exclaims, "I get queasy and feel like fainting whenever I look at that needle!" For each patient, address the following three questions:

- o What other assessment data would you like to know about the patient?
- o What therapeutic communication techniques would you use to obtain the needed assessment information?
- o How would you customize the goals, objectives, teaching strategies, and evaluation methods for each patient?

References

1. Fosbinder, D: Patient perceptions of nursing care: An emerging theory of interpersonal competence. Journal of Advanced Nursing *20*:1085, 1994.
2. Knowles, MS: The Modern Practice of Adult Education: From Pedagogy to Androgogy. Association Press, Wilton, CT, 1980.
3. Hanson, M, and Fisher, JC: Patient-centered teaching from theory to practice. American Journal of Nursing *98*(1):56, 1998.
4. London, F: Improving compliance: What you can do. RN January:43, 1998.
5. Piaget, J, and Garcia, M: Understanding Causality. WW Norton, New York, 1974.
6. Cirone, NR: Teach your children well. Nursing98 *28*(3):32hn14, 1998.
7. Katz, JR:. Providing effective patient teaching. American Journal of Nursing *97*(5):33, 1997.
8. London, F: Return demonstrations: How to validate patient education. Nursing97 *27*(2):32j, 1997.
9. Huey, R, et al: Discharge planning: Good planning means fewer hospitalizations for the chronically ill. Nursing *81*, 11–20, 1981.

Using the Problem-Solving Process To Help Patients and Families Make Decisions

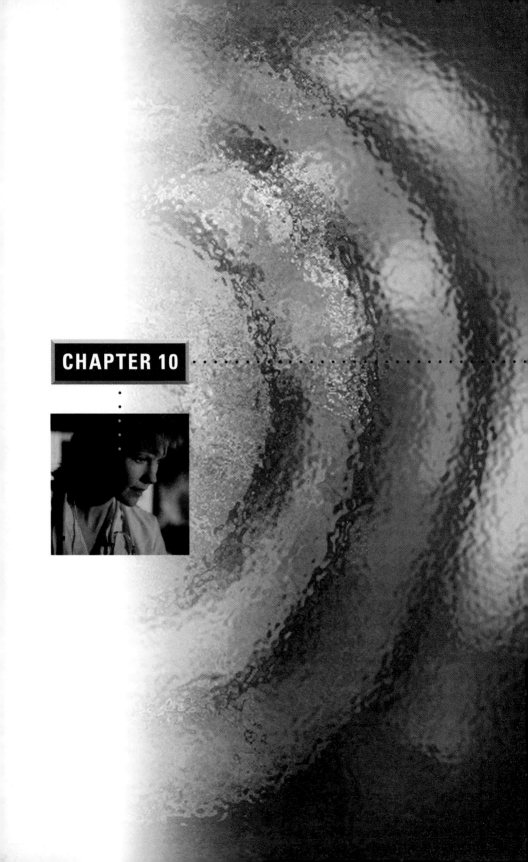

CHAPTER 10

Using the Problem-Solving Process To Help Patients and Families Make Decisions

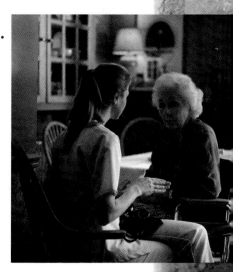

Chapter Objectives

AFTER READING THIS CHAPTER,
YOU WILL BE ABLE TO:

1. Describe the relationship between therapeutic communication and problem solving.
2. Describe each step of the problem-solving process.
3. Describe how to criticize effectively behavior.
4. Relate the problem-solving process to the nursing process.
5. Describe how to negotiate effectively an agreement to work toward mutual goals.

THIS LAST CHAPTER FOCUSES ON A VERY IMPORTANT APPLICATION OF therapeutic communication: problem solving. Specifically, you can help patients and families see problems clearly, examine their options to solve those problems, and make plans to solve problems using therapeutic communication techniques. As described in previous chapters, you must use therapeutic techniques to encourage the patient and family to ventilate and talk to you about anything that's bothering them.

Let's suppose you develop a therapeutic relationship with a patient and family, and you get them to talk openly with you about what is really bothering them. You used many therapeutic communication techniques to get them to open up and talk to you. You may have used empathy, touch, humor, and many of the basic verbal facilitating techniques described in Chapter 4. You found out what is bothering them, from their perspective. They perceive that there is a problem, and you believe you understand the nature of the problem. So now what do you do? The answer is to help them solve the problem by making logical decisions.

Basic Steps in the Problem-Solving Process

The steps in the problem-solving process originated in the field of business management in the early 1900s. Problem solving has since been applied across all disciplines, including nursing. There are eight general steps in the problem-solving process including identifying a general problem, searching out information about the problem, identifying options, examining the pros and cons of each option, choosing an option, developing a plan, implementing the plan, and evaluating results.[1]

THE GENERAL PROBLEM

Naturally, the first step in solving a problem is to identify that something's wrong. For example, say the school nurse finds a 14-year-old boy crying in the school office while waiting to see the principal. The nurse offers him tissues, touches his arm, and asks him to come into the clinic examination room to wait, realizing that it would be appropriate to provide him some privacy because he's crying. The nurse waits for him to control his crying and asks, "What happened?"

The nurse moves slowly, her voice calm and quiet as she speaks. The nurse has done well so far in using therapeutic communication techniques.[2]

The student levels with her and says tearfully, "I got caught cheating on a math test and my folks are going to kill me!" At this point, the nurse and student have identified two general problems. First, he got caught cheating. Second, his folks are going to kill him.

The nurse might like to say, "You deserve whatever punishment you get. Cheating is dishonest and despicable, and under no circumstances should cheating be tolerated." However, that would be a blaming and a spontaneous response that is certainly not therapeutic. Instead, the nurse uses empathy and says, "You must have really wanted to do well on that test. A good grade must really mean a lot to you." Remember empathy? Even though you think cheating is dishonest and intolerable, use empathy when people tell you their problem as they see it. Accept the behaviors and respond in a nonjudgmental manner. Acceptance doesn't mean that you agree with the behavior. Instead, you're trying to respond to the person's feelings and values, and arrive at what's really important to the person. You must come up with a verbal empathic response, so choose your words carefully.

SEARCHING OUT INFORMATION

An empathic response should be useful in encouraging the child to expand on what happened and why he was cheating. Although it may be tempting, the nurse wouldn't say, "Why were you cheating?" That would put the student on the defensive. Instead, the nurse made an empathic statement. The boy responded with, "My parents expect me to get an A in every class I take. If I don't get an A, I get grounded. I didn't have enough time to study like I should have because I was playing a computer game last night and I lost track of time. I swear I'll never cheat again as long as I live."

Now the nurse may be wondering, what's wrong with these parents, expecting this kid to get As in everything. So she asks, "Your parents expect an A in each course or they ground you? That sounds like a lot of pressure on you." With this communication technique, the nurse is seeking clarification and continuing to offer empathy. The boy answers, "Yeah, they expect an A or I'm grounded." The nurse says, "And you also said that you were playing computer games instead of studying." He said, "Yeah."

Next, the nurse summarizes by saying, "I see a few problems here. One is that it's not realistic to expect an A in everything. Even Einstein got a few bad grades in school." Here, a little humor can help to lighten the situation. "Second, studying has to take priority over playing on the computer. And third, cheating is something you can't wiggle out of. You'll get a zero on the test and a disciplinary warning, and your parents will be notified." He nods tearfully. At this point, the nurse and the boy have clearly identified the elements of the situation. His parents are a part of the problem, his study habits are part of the problem, and cheating is part of the problem.

EXAMINING THE OPTIONS

Next the nurse says, "You've got to go into the principal's office and talk with him about these problems. Would you like to talk to the principal by yourself, or would you like me to go into the office with you?" Going to see the principal is not an option in this situation. But whether or not the nurse goes with him is an option.

DISCUSSING THE PROS AND CONS

Next, they discuss the pros and cons of each option. The boy states, "If you go with me, what good would that do?" The nurse answers, "I can help clearly state what the problems are as we have done just now, and you wouldn't have to face him alone." She adds, "However, maybe you would prefer to go by yourself, tell him what you told me just now, and face him on your own. It's up to you to decide what you would prefer. Either way is fine with me."

CHOOSING AN OPTION

The boy states, "I think I want you to go with me." At this point, the boy has made a decision. It's very important to let the patient make the choice whenever there's a choice to be made. It's the patient's right to decide.

DEVELOPING A PLAN

The nurse says, "I think it would be best if you explained everything to him just as you did to me, and I'll be there to back you up and clarify as needed." He says, "Okay." The nurse's goal is to let this young person be as independent as possible in this situation but to back him up as needed to clearly present the situation. Sometimes a plan can be very formal, and you would develop goals and specific objectives on paper. The teaching plan as described in Chapter 9 is an example of a formal plan with goals and objectives that is used to solve the problem of a knowledge deficit.

IMPLEMENTING THE PLAN

The nurse goes with the boy into the principal's office, and the boy does well presenting the situation. The nurse needs to help only a little bit to summarize the problem clearly while the student talks to the principal.

EVALUATING ITS EFFECTS

Going with the boy was supportive and helped make sure his problems were clearly presented. At this point, the nurse could excuse herself to go and see another student who had come to her office with a stomachache.

You may be thinking at this point: This boy's problems are not solved. He's still got a problem with his parents, his study habits, and cheating. Remember, however, that these problems were not the nurse's to solve. The school psychologist, the school guidance counselor, the parents, and principal can take it from there. It's their job to figure out what to do with these problems, examine the options, look at the pros and cons, make decisions, implement them, and evaluate them. Problem solving is an ongoing process. Day in and day out, nurses solve problems and refer problems to be solved by others as appropriate.

Problems with Problem Solving

The biggest problem with problem solving is that most people don't search out enough information about the problem. They don't do enough of an assessment. They try to solve a problem without really knowing all the details. In the example, if you only examine the surface problem, the boy cheated. A simple problem, if you just look at the surface. Therefore, he gets a zero on the test, has a disciplinary warning in his file, and the offense is reported to his parents. But what about the parents putting pressure on him to get As in every course? And what about his study habits?

A thorough assessment of the problem of cheating using therapeutic communication yielded an accurate description of the cause of the problem. Once you have knowledge of the cause of the problem, then chances are much better that you can come up with more options to examine to solve problems, make good decisions, and make better plans to deal with the problem.

As comically depicted on page 247, the second biggest problem with problem solving is that people don't spend enough time examining options. You need to find out what the options are, and then spend time thinking about them. Don't rush to make a decision. Ask the advice of those who know the most about possible solutions. Regarding the parents in the situation who believe the child should have all As or be punished, the principal, school psychologist, and guidance counselor will need to develop options to handle this situation.

Many times in problem solving in nursing situations, once you have discovered the details of a problem and the circumstances that caused the problem, you tell the patient, "Now that we know what the problem is, we need to check out all the options for solving it. I know that the social worker (or occupational therapist, or physical therapist, or pharmacist, or whoever) can help shed some light on what we could possibly do about this problem. We've got to play this game with a full deck of cards. Let me do some checking, and I'll get back with you."

As you look for options, be creative. Another name for creativity in looking at options is brainstorming. Brainstorming means you can freely speak your mind about what an option might be without being criticized. Don't say things like, "That's a stupid idea" or "That will never work" when engaged in a brainstorming session. Everyone should feel free to throw out ideas that might help solve a problem. You might think that someone's idea is stupid and won't work, you just won't say it out loud in a therapeutic mode of communication. Also, although it may be okay to react spontaneously with, "That won't work!" when you're with a friend in a social situation, you shouldn't do it with a patient. Help the patient think his ideas through by discussing the pros and cons of each option. Clearly and assertively state why you think an option is good or bad and actively listen to the patient's point of view.

After looking carefully at options, the next step is making a decision. The patient and family must make a choice about one of the options. You've discussed the pros and cons of keeping the patient at home or sending him to a nursing home, for example. The family decided to take the patient home. You've done nothing to influence the decision. You've simply given the options and discussed them. The patient and family have the right to decide what is best for them.

In another example, say a patient has a problem with smoking and you've explained smoking cessation and discussed the options of a nicotine patch, self-help tapes, and smoking cessation classes offered at the American Lung Association. In this case, the patient did not choose any of the options and kept on smoking. You might think the patient didn't make a decision, but you'd be wrong. The patient's decision was to do nothing about the problem. Doing nothing is also a de-

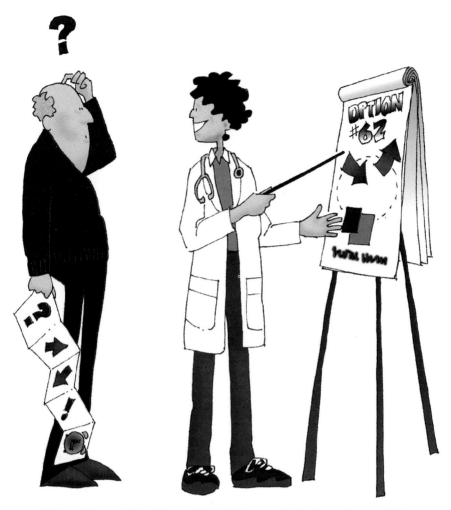

One of the problems with problem solving is that people don't spend enough time examining options.

cision. You may not agree with the decision, but the patient has the right to choose *or not to choose* the options that you believe will lead to a more optimal state of health.

Much of the time, nurses end up developing and implementing a teaching plan once the patient or family has made the decision. For example, if the family chooses to take the patient home instead of sending him to a nursing home, a teaching plan will be developed to teach the patient and family self-care in the home, as was described in Chapter 9.

Then imagine that this happens: You've done your best to teach the patient and family self-care at home, but they call back in 2 weeks and say that they just can't handle the patient at home, as much as they would have liked to. They've evaluated the situation, things aren't working out, and they decide to try another option. They decide to put the patient in a nursing home. The problem is now to find a suitable nursing home. Now you give the family the options on types of nursing homes in the area and look at the pros and cons of each. Then they decide which one would be best. Next, plans are made between the nurses at the home and the family for when the patient will move to the nursing home. The family and patient continue to evaluate the situation as the patient moves into the nursing home.

Many health care providers of varying specialties may work with the same patient and family on the same problem. So you need to know what your piece of the problem is and what you need to help the patient and family resolve. You may be involved in discovering what the problem really is. You may be involved in giving and discussing options. But you (or any other health care provider) may not be involved in every stage of problem solving for every problem. Although you may be involved in many steps of the problem-solving process, it's important to remember that the patient and family must decide for themselves during the decision-making phase of problem solving, with your support for their decision.

Handling a "Bad" Decision

Sometimes, although the patient and family members make a decision based on the information available to them, the solution doesn't work out for the best. Perhaps there were repercussions that were not anticipated at the time of the decision. In some instances, nurses also make bad decisions and have negative results from those decisions. What should you do, and what should you advise a patient or family member to do, when it becomes apparent that a decision isn't working out?

Even the most reasoned decisions can still be perceived by others as a big mistake. If this situation occurs and you now realize that you didn't consider all the ramifications of the decision, you must apologize, accept responsibility, and offer a solution. For example, say, "I'm sorry, I realize now that my decision was wrong. At the time, it seemed like the best course of action in my professional opinion. In the future though, I will. . . ."

Swallowing your pride and admitting that you were wrong will earn the respect of those around you. Nobody's perfect, and everyone recognizes that bad decisions happen. Work to correct the decision, if possible. You also need to forgive yourself for the bad decision and let it go. Sometimes making the wrong decision isn't entirely bad if you grow and learn as a result of the mistake.[3]

Responding to
Unacceptable Behavior

The cheating behavior described earlier in the chapter is definitely unacceptable behavior, but it is not your problem to solve. With patients and family members, however, you may sometimes need to criticize a behavior. Remember to use therapeutic communication techniques as you tell someone that they've done something wrong.[4]

For example, consider the patient who seems always to be late for her appointments at the prenatal clinic. You let it go twice because she had a good excuse both times, but this is the third time it happened and you want to say something about it. She has the last appointment of the day, and you've been getting home late because of her tardiness. Use the following suggestions to frame your conversation.

Begin the conversation with something positive. Don't greet the person with criticism or displeasure. Something general, like "How are you doing today?" or "How are things going?" are positive opening queries. From these positive open-ended questions, you can get a general impression of the patient's emotional state. If things are evidently going fairly well, and you don't detect another problem that should take higher priority, then you can begin the criticism.

To do so, criticize the specific act, not the person. Say something like, "I need to discuss a problem with you. This is the third appointment in a row for which you've been late." Don't say, "You're always late," which is too sweeping a generality. Also don't say, "You're always late and inconsiderate of others," which now moves into name-calling. However, you may want to add something about the consequences of her behavior to your statement. For example, you might say, "As a result of your lateness, we've had to keep the office open longer than our scheduled hours." Keep it short and to the point. Don't lecture.

Also, make sure that the behavior you criticize can indeed be changed. Although you may think that the patient should be able to arrive at her appointments on time, suppose she can't leave work early enough to do so, she has babysitter problems, or there are other problems beyond her control. She may have a good reason and something that can't be changed about her situation.

In your conversation, make sure that the other person understands the reason for your criticism. Tell her about having to keep the office open beyond its scheduled closing or that you've been late getting home to your family. Again, keep this short and to the point, without giving a lecture.

Throughout your discussion, use therapeutic communication skills. Use "I" and "we" as you attempt to work out the problem. Stress that you want to work out the problem together by looking at the surrounding circumstances and options. Show the person that you understand her feelings by using empathy as she describes the problem from her perspective. Don't threaten the person by saying something like, "If you're late next time, we won't let you in the clinic." And don't use sarcasm by saying something like, "Hey, it's about time you showed up. What's the excuse today?"

Finally, engage the patient in the problem-solving process. To do so, ask the patient what makes it hard for her to get to her appointment at its scheduled 4 pm time. Maybe she'll say something like, "My mother babysits for me and she can't leave work until 4 o'clock." So look for other options. Find out whether the patient can come at another time of day. Find out whether she can bring her children with her and have your receptionist keep an eye on them. Find out if anyone else can watch them. As you examine each option, let the patient decide which one suits her best. Then make a plan, implement the plan, and evaluate the results. Don't offer what you can't accept: that she continues to come late for her appointments.[2]

Problem Solving and the Nursing Process

The problem-solving process is the foundation of the nursing process. The nursing process involves learning to perform assessments, making nursing diagnoses, developing a plan of care, implementing the plan of care, and evaluating the effects of the plan of care. Each of these steps parallels the steps of the problem-solving process.

ASSESSMENT

As a nurse, you'll spend a great deal of time assessing patients and families. You'll do physical assessments, emotional assessments, environmental assessments, and cultural assessments. For example, consider the patient who had a bowel resection 2 days ago. You're assigned to take care of him on this particular clinical day. You know the general problem: He had surgery on his bowel because he had an abdominal abscess and a bowel obstruction. The biopsy report indicates that he has cancer of the bowel.

The first thing you do is an in-depth assessment of applicable physical, psychological, social, and cultural parameters, and you obtain a database. To obtain the database, you gather information about the person's health state that's relevant to the provision of nursing care.

Here's some of the assessment data from the database that you'll need for this patient. The patient has an abdominal wound and dressing, and he's getting morphine every 3 hours as needed. His temperature is 100.5°F, he has two drains with purulent drainage and fecal material in the drains, and his white blood cell count is 12.9. He is permitted nothing by mouth, has a nasogastric tube draining his stomach, and has an intravenous line through which he's receiving fluids and total parenteral nutrition. He's on bed rest and can sit in a chair if two assistants help him move. He is 5'10" and weighs 139 pounds, his hemoglobin is 10, and he's lethargic and fatigued. He fidgets with his hands and says that he's nervous. He cries and says he knows that he's going to die. He says that his back and his wound hurt very badly.

NURSING DIAGNOSIS

The nursing diagnosis is actually the summary statement about the assessment findings. Nurses label the problem and add a careful description of the problem that includes evidence that support the finding of a problem. Nurses focus on priority problems that they'll address on a particular day. In the case of this patient, the problems can be summarized as:

- Pain from surgery, a wound, and morphine every 3 hours as needed
- Infection from the abscess, purulent and fecal drainage, a high white blood cell count, and a fever
- Nutritional problems from receiving nothing by mouth, a nasogastric tube, an intravenous line for total parenteral nutrition, anemia from low hemoglobin, and a low weight of 139 pounds for a person who's 5'10" tall
- Patient is anxious as evidenced by fidgeting, crying, and verbalizing that he's nervous and knows he's going to die
- Reduced mobility and a high risk for falling from bed rest, plexipulses (sequential compression devices), many tubes to trip over, lethargy, and pain medications.

Nursing diagnoses that you would use to cover these problems, as put forth by the North American Nursing Diagnosis Association, include the following:

- Pain
- Impaired Skin Integrity
- Risk for Altered Body Temperature
- Risk for Infection
- Altered Nutrition: Less than Body Requirements

- Fatigue
- Anxiety
- Impaired Physical Mobility.[5]

Sometimes students get too caught up in putting the appropriate nursing diagnosis labels on problems. It's much better to have an accurate description and assessment of a situation than to worry so much about the exact label.

PLANNING

For each problem identified, you need to figure out options for solving it and then document them in a nursing care plan. First, write goals and patient behavioral objectives that you hope will be attained. For example, one general goal will be to control pain. The patient behavioral objectives will be to verbalize that he is comfortable, that his pain is no worse than 1 or 2 on a scale of 0 to 10, in which 0 is no pain and 10 is the worst pain imaginable. Another behavioral objective may be that the patient will move about in bed and perform range-of-motion exercises without wincing or reporting pain.

Next, figure out nursing interventions that may alleviate the pain. Carefully consider all options. One option may be to offer pain medications every 3 hours to stay ahead of the pain. Consider the pros and cons of pain medication; for example, you don't want the patient to become addicted, but you do want to control pain. Other options may be to offer visual imagery, relaxation exercises, or a back massage for relaxation and reduction of the backache. Another pain-control option may be to use therapeutic touch and to hold the patient's hand as you talk with him. The pros and cons are that some, but not all, patients respond to these nonpharmacologic pain management techniques. You'll need to find the right combination of techniques to control pain in each patient.

For each identified nursing diagnosis, you'll write goals and objectives and you'll consider the pros and cons of options used for nursing interventions. In this example, goals, objectives, and nursing interventions were described for pain control only. In developing a comprehensive care plan, you would of course develop goals, objectives, and interventions for each nursing diagnosis.

IMPLEMENTATION

Implementation is the time spent in interacting with the patient and performing nursing interventions that will meet his goals and objectives. Implementation is similar to problem solving in that you must explain to the patient the options and give him choices regarding control of pain. Let's assume that you and the patient have a mutual goal of pain control. Now you and the patient need to figure out how to accomplish this goal. Does the patient want injections of medication? Does the patient want a back massage? Does the patient want to try visual imagery or relaxation exercises? You wouldn't ask the patient if he wants therapeutic touch; this is something that you'd try and watch the response. Does he pull away or cling to your hand?

EVALUATION

The final step in both problem solving and the nursing process is evaluation. Specifically, were the goals and objectives met? Were the interventions effective to alleviate the patient's pain? Sometimes goals and objectives weren't realistic and need to be modified. An optimist would say, "You didn't fail; you just need to redesign the goals and objectives!" Seriously, however, sometimes your plan may not have been realistic.

Suppose you go to take care of this patient, and the patient is soon feeling much better. The nasogastric tube was removed during the evening, after you performed the assessment and went home to develop your plan of care. The patient was sitting up, sipping clear liquids, and looking much better by 7 am when you came in, and he only required one injection for pain during the night. Pain would no longer be a prime consideration in the care of this patient, although it would still be a problem. Infection control and wound care might end up to be the priority problem of the day.

As you develop a plan for infection control, you would plan to provide wound care and also to provide general hygiene by helping the patient bathe. You need to perform a sterile dressing change, of course, but you also realize that any secretions on his skin can contribute to skin breakdown and infection. You also realize that he would feel a lot more comfortable and probably experience less pain if he's clean and feeling fresh. You go into the room to update your assessment and then tell the patient, "I'll get the items together to help with your bath." But the patient says, "I'm too tired for a bath today. I just want to lie here and watch TV." It's time to do problem solving using negotiation skills to establish mutual goals.

Negotiate To Solve Problems and Establish Mutual Goals

This patient doesn't want a bath because he's tired and wants to relax. You think he needs a bath to control infection and promote comfort. It's time to negotiate using therapeutic communication techniques. Negotiations are something that we do every day of our lives. In nursing, we negotiate with patients, families, and other health care providers using therapeutic communication techniques. You must learn to confront and negotiate differences using therapeutic communication techniques.[6]

There are two basic forms of negotiation. There is a traditional model, in which you would take a position, defend and argue the position, and then make concessions and compromise.[7] In the example, you might say, "You have to take a bath this morning to help prevent germs from getting in your wound."

In return, he might say, with increased volume and agitation, "I just told you I don't want a bath. The wound is covered and germs can't get in. I'm tired and I want to relax."

You might argue back, also growing upset that he doesn't believe you when you said he needed the bath to prevent infection, "When I uncover the wound to change the dressing, germs can get in. Everything in the surrounding environment, including you, needs to be clean to prevent infection."

He says, "I want to rest now, come back later to do the bath."

You say, "I can wait only an hour because I have another patient who also needs a bath."

The patient says, "Okay, boy, you drive a hard bargain. Just leave me alone for now!"

The problem with this form of negotiation is that it strains relationships. Even if you do come back in an hour, you'll probably meet some resistance then also because there's a conflict between you and the patient. A "win-lose" attitude develops, with each of you tied personally to the problem.[8] The patient may be thinking, "How dare she tell me what I have to do?" You may be thinking, "This patient is very uncooperative and doesn't believe I know what I'm doing when I tell him he has to take a bath to prevent infection." If you do find yourself getting angry, and there are times when everyone does, take steps to cool down. You can always say, "Let me think about this situation for a few minutes" and excuse yourself from the room to think about what happened and how to proceed from this point.[2]

A more therapeutic approach to negotiations is based on a special form of problem solving called interest-based bargaining.[7] The steps in the interest-based bargaining approach are outlined in the following section. They're firmly rooted in the basic problem-solving process and therapeutic communication skills.

FOCUS ON ISSUES, NOT PERSONALITIES

The general problem in the scenario just described is that you want to assist the patient with a bath and the patient doesn't want one. You insist, "You have to have one" and the patient responds with, "I told you I don't want one." The interchange becomes a personality power clash. Instead, as soon as the patient said, "I'm too tired for a bath and I want to relax," you should have used some empathy and humor. You could have said, "You've been through a lot with surgery and everything else we've been doing to you the last few days. We've really beaten up on you!" His response would have been, "You can say that again," with a smile.

IDENTIFY INTERESTS RATHER THAN FORMULATING POSITIONS

By using this principle, you let the patient know that you want what he wants. You could say, "I'm concerned about your wound and about keeping germs from entering it when I change the dressing. The sooner we get this wound healed up, the sooner you can get home." His response would have been, "I want out of here as soon as possible, whatever you need to do to get this wound healed, just do it."

DEVELOP AND FOLLOW OBJECTIVE STANDARDS

You and the patient have now agreed that getting the wound to heal and getting home are the top priorities. Next, you could say, "To keep germs out of the wound, everything in the environment needs to be clean, including you. That's why a bath is a very important part of your care, although I can see that you're tired this morning." He says, " I didn't realize how important a bath was, but I am very tired." The objective standard is that the environment and everything in it (including the patient) must be kept clean to prevent infection. You and the patient have agreed on this standard.

CREATE OPTIONS TO SATISFY INTERESTS

To help the patient decide in favor of a bath, you could offer him pleasant options. For example, you might say, "I could help with your bath if you're too tired to do it yourself, and you could watch TV while we do it together. You could rest after that." Another option would be, " I could come back in an hour if you'd prefer to get some rest right now."

EVALUATE EACH OPTION TO DETERMINE WHETHER IT MEETS THE STANDARD THAT WAS SET

In response to your options, the patient says, "Well, I appreciate the offer to help me do it, but I am very tired. If you don't mind coming back in an hour, that would be terrific."

AGREE ON SOLUTIONS THAT MEET STANDARDS BEST

The nurse says, "No problem, I've got another patient who also needs help with a bath. I'll help her first and then come back and help you." He says, "I'll see you in an hour." And in an hour, he'll probably be ready for a bath.

By using this process, you and the patient agreed on a goal of preventing infection in the wound. You also agreed that a bath is very important to prevent infection. In addition, the patient has become a partner in his care, he's motivated to have a bath, and he appears to be much more willing to cooperate in attaining a mutual goal.

All you've done is rearrange the elements of the previous argument by using interest-based bargaining and focusing on mutual gains in the situation. You've shown respect for the patient and focused on the long-term view of how things will improve after reaching a solution.[2] Specifically, the wound will heal and the patient can get home faster.

SUMMARY

It's very important that you understand the problem-solving process and apply it to the nursing care of patients. Both the nursing process and the process of interest-based negotiations to establish mutual goals are firmly rooted in the problem-solving process. In that process, you'll identify a general problem, gather information about the problem, examine options for addressing the problem, discuss the pros and cons of each option, decide to choose an option or to let things continue as they are, develop a plan, implement the plan, and evaluate whether the plan was effective.

Nurses use the problem-solving process and therapeutic communication techniques to criticize unacceptable behavior. You must begin by saying something positive. Then criticize the specific act, not the person. Make sure it's possible for the patient to change the behavior and that the patient understands the reason for your criticism. Then you can initiate the problem-solving process. The general problem is the unacceptable behavior, so search out information about what causes that behavior. Next, look for options, discuss them, form a plan, implement it, and evaluate it. As you work with the patient to solve the problem of unacceptable behavior, use general therapeutic communication techniques.

The problem-solving process is the basis for the nursing process, which includes five steps. The first step involves assessing the patient and family; this equates to searching out information about patient problems in the problem-solving process. The second step involves correctly sorting out the assessment information, grouping the information under diagnostic labels, and making nursing diagnoses. The third step involves developing a nursing plan of care that includes goals, objections, and nursing interventions that are options of care. The fourth step involves implementing the plan of care and involves negotiating goals, objectives, and interventions with patients, giving them options, and letting them decide what's best for them. The last step involves evaluating whether the plan was effective to meet the goals and objectives.

Nurses must become skilled at negotiation to establish mutual goals with patients and to avoid conflict. Interest-based negotiation is based on principles of problem solving and therapeutic communication. You must learn to focus on issues, not personalities; identify interests rather than formulate positions; develop and follow objective standards; create options to satisfy interests; evaluate each option to determine whether or not it meets the standards that were set; and agree on solutions that best meet the standards.

COMMUNICATION EXERCISES

1 The following are problem situations loosely based on real-life examples. Develop an initial response to each problem situation using principles of therapeutic communication and problem solving.

o Mrs. Rebecca Bennington is a 26-year-old attractive and vivacious secretary at the bank across the street from the clinic. One day, on her lunch hour, she came into the clinic to have a small, pain-less ulcer on her upper lip examined. A culture of the sore was taken and she was instructed to come back in 3 days to get the results of her test and to determine the appropriate treatment based on test results. At her appointment, she was informed by the physician that the ulcer was a chancre sore caused by syphilis and that her husband would also need treatment. You go into the room to give her additional information on syphilis. She is crying and says, "I've been married for over 6 years to my husband and have never cheated on him. How could he do this to me? I don't want to talk to him, and I don't even want to look at him." What should you say and do next?

o Mr. Pinkerton is a 47-year-old, socially prominent accountant who was admitted to the outpatient clinic three times in the last 6 months for treatment for accidents sustained by passing out after drinking too much. On this admission, he broke his hand after falling during a drinking episode. He is witty and cooperative, and willingly participates in Alcoholics Anonymous group meetings at the clinic. You are the group leader at the Alcoholics Anonymous meeting, and he comes over to talk with you after the meeting and jokes with you about the help he needs opening doors, dressing, and other activities that require the use of his broken hand. He says that his hands shake from "bottle fatigue." His hands shake as he pours himself a drink of water, and he becomes visibly upset as he soaks his shirt while attempting to take a drink. What should you say and do next?

o Miss Amanda Severt is 35 years old and is being treated for an overactive thyroid. Your assessment reveals that she is weak and tired, and has lost 30 pounds. She is 5'6" and weighs 110 pounds, even though she eats an enormous amount of food. She is taking medication, but you would like to teach her about increasing her calorie intake to gain weight. You are to provide nutritional teaching. Where do you start?

2 As a class activity to practice therapeutic techniques and problem solving, role play the above-mentioned situations in front of the class. One student can be the nurse, the other student can be the patient, and the interaction can be evaluated by the entire class. As an option, the role playing could be videotaped and the resulting video stopped and started to review and focus on different parts of the interaction.

References

1. Chenevert, M: Pro-Nurse Handbook. Mosby, St. Louis, 1985.
2. Anderson, K: 16 tips for reaching agreement. Nursing98 *28*(7):64, 1998.
3. Grensing-Pophal, L: Whoops! Now what? Nursing98 *28*(1):64, 1998.
4. North Eastern Ohio Education Association: 12 ways to criticize effectively. News and Views *27*(7):5, 1998.
5. North American Nursing Diagnosis Association: Nursing Diagnoses: Definitions & Classification 1999. Philadelphia, Author.
6. Sharf, BF: Teaching patients to speak up: Past and future trends. Patient education Counseling *11*:95, 1988.
7. Fisher, R, and Ury, W: Getting to Yes: Negotiating Agreement Without Giving in, ed 2. Penguin Books, New York, 1991.
8. Hendricks, W: How to Manage Conflict. National Press Publications, Shawnee Mission, Kansas, 1991.

Index

. . . .

Page numbers followed by *f* indicate figures.

Behavior (*continued*)
  effect of hormones on, 40
  gender differences in nonverbal,
    53–54
  patient decision not to change,
    236–237
  psychomotor, 236
  responding to unacceptable,
    249–250
Behavioral capabilities, 214
Belonging, 18
Biological influences on gender
    communication, 40–41
Birth and infancy, 197–198
Blamer as communication style,
    20–21, 66, 68, 71, 120
Blaming, 65
Body image and self-esteem, 73–75,
    90
Body language
  and nurses, 54
  observing, in therapeutic
    communication, 12–13
  and responding to messages, 14
Brain sex test, 55–56*f*
Brainstorming, 246
Burnout, preventing, 111, 112*f*

Care, patient participation in,
    123–125
Catecholamines, release of, in
    arousal phase, 19, 178
Challenging statements, 105–106
Childhood, 198
Children, learning in, 216–217
Clarifying, 109
Clothing colors and styles, 76
Cognitive knowledge, 213, 234
Cognitive objectives, 233–234
Color analysis, 75–76
Communication
  assertive/responsive competence
    patterns in, 127–131*f*
  breaking through barriers to
    successful, 119–141
  competence scale for, 140*f*
  definition of, 5, 6
  difficulties in, 131
  distortion factors in, 17–19
  effects of self-esteem and body
    image on, 63–83
  elements of, 5*f*
  emotional responses in, 19–20

evaluating skills in, 25–26*f*
factors in successful, 5–6
gender differences in, 31–59
identifying patterns of verbal and
    nonverbal, 33–34, 39–41
and low self-esteem, 66, 68
messages in, 4–6
nurse-patient, 7–10, 8*f*
in nursing, 70–71
physical responses in, 19–20
in professional relationships,
    10–12
therapeutic, 7–15, 125–131,
    211–237
Communication theory, 4–6
Complaining, 138–139, 141
Compliments, 53
Computer, as communication style,
    22, 66, 68, 71
Concerns, focusing immediate, first,
    215
Confidentiality, patient, 50–51
Conflict, 46
Congruent leveler, 69–70
Contact, making, with patient,
    185–186
Convalescence, 94
Conversational rituals, 52–53
Cooperative overlapping, versus
    talking alone, 47–48
Crying. *See also* Tears
  nontherapeutic responses to,
    194–195
  by nurses, 206–207
  therapeutic responses to, 203–
    205
Cultural barriers, 222–223
Culture
  assessment of feelings on, 35–38*f*
  beliefs on, 34
  effects of, on patient assessment,
    229
  influence on gender
    communications, 34, 39–40

Death, 200
Decision, handling bad, 248–249
Defense mechanisms, 222. *See also*
    Denial; Rationalization
Defensiveness, 107
Denial, 93, 94, 99, 222
Denying statements, 105–106
Dependency, 96–97

Hostility, open, 132–134
Hugging, 160–162
Humor. *See also* Laughter
  in avoidance tactics, 183–184
  criteria for determining appropriateness of, in psychotherapeutic relationships, 179*f*
  definition of, 175–176
  in embarrassing situations, 182
  encouraging emotional release using, 173–188
  ethnic, 177
  gender differences in using, 184–185
  making mistakes with, 188
  nontherapeutic, 177–178
  nurses' use of, 185–188
  patients use of, 181–185
  psychological effects of, 180–181
  sources of, 175*f*
  therapeutic, 174, 175–177
  in unpleasant situations, 182–183

Illness, 200
  emotional reactions to stress of, 89–112
  patient's personal and unique response to, 95–101
  physical stages of, 91, 92*f*
  psychosocial stages of, 91, 91*f*, 93
  as threat to self-esteem, 90–91
  transition to, 93
Implementation in problem solving, 252–253
Infancy, 197–198
Information
  offering, 109–110
  provider versus listener, 48–50
  searching out, 243–244
Inhibition of nursing touch, 154–155
Interest-based bargaining, 254
Interests
  creating options to satisfy, 255
  identifying, 255
Interruption and nurses, 48
Intimate zone, 157–158
Issues, focusing on, 254–255

Jewelry, 77
Joking, 53

Knowledge. *See also* Education; Learning; Teaching
  cognitive, 213
  health, 226–227

Language. *See also* Communication
  body, 12–13, 14, 54
  gender differences in, 51–53
Late adult life, 199–200
Laughter, 121. *See also* Humor
  physiological effects of, 178–180
  tips for putting, to work, 187*f*
Learner, assessing, 217
Learning. *See also* Education; Knowledge; Teaching
  basic content, 223–228
  basic principles of patient-centered, 212–214
  in children, 216–217
  evaluation and documentation of, 235–236
  factors that inhibit, 221–223
  principles of adult, 214–216
  reinforcing all, 220
  steps to facilitate, 217–221
Learning style, 231
Leveler
  as communication style, 23–24, 71
  congruent, 69–70
Leveling
  and congruent leader, 69
  and strong self-esteem, 121–122
Life Fields Theory, 17
Lifestyle, adapting teaching to, 215
Listener versus information provider, 48–50
Listening, active, 205–206
Love, 18
Low self-esteem, 64–65
  communication styles of people with, 66, 68
  and put-down humor, 177

Massage, 151–152, 163–164
Medications, 224
Messages. *See also* Communication
  elements of, 4–6
  responding to real, in therapeutic communication, 14–15
Middle age, 199
Motivation, 230–231